HOLISTIC HEALTH AND NUTRITION

A SIMPLE 11 STEP APPROACH TO HOLISTIC HEALTH WITH NUTRITION

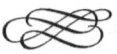

YOTA KOUYAS GERRIOR R.H.N

Holistic Health and Nutrition

An 11 Step Approach to Holistic Health With Nutrition

Yota Kouyas Gerrior R.H.N.

© Copyright 2022 - All rights reserved.

The content contained within this book may not be reproduced, duplicated or transmitted without direct written permission from the author or the publisher.

Under no circumstances will any blame or legal responsibility be held against the publisher, or author, for any damages, reparation, or monetary loss due to the information contained within this book, either directly or indirectly.

Legal Notice:

This book is copyright protected. It is only for personal use. You cannot amend, distribute, sell, use, quote or paraphrase any part, or the content within this book, without the consent of the author or publisher.

Disclaimer Notice:

Please note the information contained within this document is for educational and entertainment purposes only. All effort has been executed to present accurate, up to date, reliable, complete information. No warranties of any kind are declared or implied. Readers acknowledge that the author is not engaged in the rendering of legal, financial, medical or professional advice. The content within this book has been derived from various sources. Please consult a licensed professional before attempting any techniques outlined in this book.

By reading this document, the reader agrees that under no circumstances is the author responsible for any losses, direct or indirect, that are incurred as a result of the use of the information contained within this document, including, but not limited to, errors, omissions, or inaccuracies.

A SPECIAL GIFT TO OUR READER

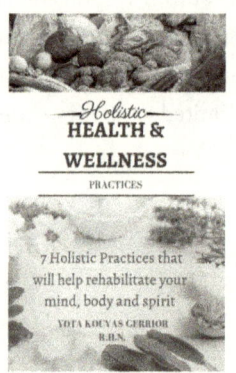

Included with your book purchase are our Holistic Health and Wellness Practices. These simple practices will give you seven easy steps towards achieving Holistic Health and Wellness.

Click on the link below and let us know which email address to deliver it to.

www.yotasholistichealth.com

INTRODUCTION

People don't understand this: our bodies are impacted by what we eat. So it's not enough to focus on the texture and flavour of the food, even though the anticipation and enthusiasm help us enjoy our food. But prioritizing the nutrients, they provide over their caloric content is what our bodies truly need to stay healthy.

So many things, including our food choices, influence our health. If you constantly feed your body with healthy foods, you'll feel much better than when your diet is made up of unhealthy foods. It can sometimes be challenging to find the time to prepare healthy meals, especially when you live a busy

INTRODUCTION

lifestyle. No one wants to return from a long day of work to begin to cook a meal that may take an hour or two to get ready. It's easier to grab an already made meal. But these foods aren't usually beneficial to our health.

We live in a world of unavoidable stress. The demands of life never seem to end. As a result, we put so much pressure on our bodies just to meet our day-to-day commitments and responsibilities. In the process, we forget to properly nourish our bodies and seek the nearest vending machine when our stress levels are high.

Many of us struggle to differentiate between a poor diet and a healthy diet. My rule of thumb is that if your grandparents wouldn't recognize a food, it probably is unhealthy. The unfortunate part of eating unhealthy food is that it initially makes us feel relaxed, but it is short-lived. Junk foods worsen our stress levels, leading to problems like fatigue and insomnia. So under chronic stress, recognizing the connection between our overall well-being and nutrition creates better opportunities to optimize living a healthier life.

This book will serve as a guideline for

INTRODUCTION

anyone intending to cultivate a holistic approach to care. It's not like orthodox medicine doesn't work because it does. We use it to treat diseases and illnesses, using different treatment methods. Likewise, conventional medicine solely focuses on treating the symptoms we display and not necessarily other confounding factors. But holistic health is the total opposite. It's aimed at enhancing our body's ability to help itself. So as you read through each chapter, you'll get a deeper understanding of holistic health and nutrition.

The human body is a highly complex structure consisting of different systems, cells, and organs that work together to keep us alive. Each structure has a specific role it plays in the body. For instance, our eyes are responsible for our sight. However, it works together with our brain, the nervous, muscular, and circulatory systems to support its role. The same can be said about other organs in our bodies. For example, the brain helps interpret what our eyes are seeing while the muscular system acts as a muscle tissue that allows our eyes to rotate and turn in its socket. The circulatory system supplies blood and nutrients to our eyes, and the nervous system transmits information from our eyes to the brain.

The nutrients in our food enable these structures in our bodies to perform their necessary function. Suppose an essential nutrient is absent, aspects of function and our health decline. By reading this book, you'll understand the link between nutrition and health, which will guide your decision-making and help you become an informed consumer. This is especially important if you live a busy lifestyle. You'll be able to tame your stress levels as you begin to choose healthier options. In turn, you'll have more energy to fuel your daily activities, and the quality of your sleep will improve.

As you read this book, you'll learn:

- What holistic health and nutrition is.
- The body systems, functions, and importance in living a healthy lifestyle with proper nutrients to help aid these systems.
- Steps on making your body feel its best, with techniques on how and

INTRODUCTION

what nutrients your body needs to accomplish this.
- Natural ways to help you beat chronic stress and fatigue to help you feel more energized.
- You'll be guided on managing your stress through a holistic approach and not medication.

I've been studying holistic health and nutritional aspects of holistic health for ten years to help with my chronic health annoyances. I received my Diploma in Natural Health and Nutrition from The Canadian School of Natural Nutrition. In addition, I earned a Diploma in Personal Training with Honors from Ashworth College. Therefore, I know the body inside and out and how nutrition can affect our health. I also received my certification as a personal trainer with Canfitpro Canada.

I love reading about holistic health and looking for remedies to aid people in day-to-day health concerns. I'm passionate about helping you overcome fatigue and stress and energize your mind, body, and spirit with a nutritional approach. This subject matters

INTRODUCTION

deeply to me because what you're about to learn can help you overcome your daily health concerns by just following a few simple techniques.

I am writing this book because I've used these simple techniques in the past to overcome many obstacles when it comes to feeling overtired, overwhelmed, and most importantly, how to deal with day-to-day stressors. I've equally used these practices to help many individuals with chronic stressors through nutritional coaching. As a result, I have learned to reverse the negative aspects of stress and move toward a more positive outlook. Looking at the positive points in everything I do, over the negative has helped me turn my view of life into the most enjoyable version it can be.

Are you ready to activate your body's health potential through nutrition? Keep reading.

HOLISTIC NUTRITION PAST, PRESENT, AND FUTURE

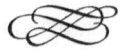

Before the agricultural revolution, our ancestors ate a diet consisting of vegetables, fruits, and meat. There was no processed food. They hunted and gathered their food. Food was a matter of what was available, which corresponded to the changing seasons—the presence and absence of certain fruits and vegetables and the migration or movement of animals.

When there was food, they walked long distances to get it, so they expended lots of energy in the process. From the way society was set up during that era, our ancestors lived a very active lifestyle. However, when the agricultural revolution emerged, our eating habits changed. Rather than living a life organized around the search for food, we could cultivate different fruits and vegetables and domesticate many animals. So there was a stable, accessible, and storable source of food.

But this changed the way we handled food, subsequently changing our diet. To extend their shelf life, we began to preserve foods by different means like canning, salting and drying. Instead of eating fresh foods, we began to process our foods. Often processing entails stripping the food of some of its nutrients. So the composition and quality of our diets changed.

The kinds of foods we eat today are very different from the diet of our ancestors. If you look around, the numbers of fast-food restaurants are continuously growing, and our health is suffering from the effects of these foods. More and more people are consuming soft drinks, pastries, chips, and so on, usually high in fat, sodium, or carbohydrate. You may feel satisfied from consuming these foods, but they aren't nutrient-dense and may not leave room for you to consume other nutritious foods.

. . .

A Holistic Nutritional Approach to Health

I use the term 'holistic' to mirror a complete system made up of different parts that are interconnected. Each component can have a significant influence on the complete system. When it comes to our health, I'm looking at how every aspect of our lives can impact our overall well-being instead of one isolated dimension of wellness. For instance, if you're suffering from clinical depression but are physically healthy, your overall health has declined because the illness may be affecting your emotional, social, or mental health.

On the other hand, nutrition nourishes your body when you consume foods. These foods meet your body's dietary needs. But nutrition can vary from person to person depending on their lifestyle, nutritional concerns, age, and gender. For instance, if you're an athlete, your diet will be different from that of a pregnant woman. Nevertheless, good nutrition is a fundamental part of good health. According to The World Health Organization (WHO), good nutrition is a combination of an adequate, well-balanced diet together with regular physical exercise (2022).

What do we gain in return? A healthy

weight from eating unprocessed foods, typically lower in calories, compared to processed, junk foods; we'll look younger; our quality of sleep will improve; our brains will function better, and the state of our minds will improve. However, bad nutrition does the opposite. It can weaken our immunity, harm our physical and mental development, increase our susceptibility to diseases, and make us less productive.

What Is Holistic Nutrition?

We can't talk about nutrition without talking about food. We need food to energize and nourish our bodies. When we eat, our food is broken down in the body, and nutrients are released in the process. Nutrients allow our bodies to function properly. Since we can't consume nutrients in isolation but only in the foods we eat, the composition of our diets influences health outcomes.

There are seven nutrients our bodies need daily for optimal health. These include fats, proteins, carbohydrates, vitamins, minerals, water, and dietary fibre.

These nutrients can be categorized into

micro and macronutrients. Macronutrients are carbohydrates, proteins, fat, dietary fibre, and water. Our bodies need these nutrients in larger quantities to function well. Micronutrients are vitamins and minerals. Our bodies need these nutrients in small amounts. Thus, a healthy diet supplies our bodies with these nutrients.

The sources of these nutrients are just as important as the quantity we consume. To ensure your diet is healthy, most of your daily calories should come from eating foods containing the following significant nutrients: fresh fruits and vegetables, whole grains, legumes, and lean protein. In contrast, foods high in salt, refined sugar, and unhealthy fats (particularly trans fat and saturated fats) should be minimized.

You should be consuming the recommended amount of these foods for your diet to be healthy. These consist of at least five servings of fruits and vegetables a day and limit our salt intake to under five grams. In addition, one should shift from consuming saturated fats to unsaturated fats, remove foods high in industrially-produced trans fats and reduce the consumption of foods containing refined sugars to under 5% of our total everyday energy intake (2022).

Every human has feelings, emotions, thoughts, and personalities. Our thoughts can trigger different physiological responses that can affect our health. If, for instance, something was bothering you emotionally, your heart rate may increase, you may sweat more, or have trouble sleeping. These physiological responses can manifest physically in the form of nausea, body pains, fatigue, and so on. So when I talk about what it means to be healthy, I'm not solely focused on the absence of physical diseases.

Our overall health comes from balancing our body, mind, and spirit working together in harmony. Sometimes when people talk about the connection between the mind, body, and spirit, the interpretation of what they mean can be confusing. But it simply refers to our physical, mental, emotional, and spiritual health. All these components of wellness affect one another and our overall health. Any imbalance among these three integral aspects of our health can make us sick.

The focus of holistic nutrition isn't just about providing our bodies with macro and micronutrients, nor is it about counting calories. Instead, it's about using natural approaches to health, such as a healthy diet and healthy lifestyle choices to balance our mind, body, and spirit to re-establish optimal health. It also involves using all-natural dietary supplements, spirituality, and other complementary practices to help protect against diseases.

Holistic nutrition looks at the body as a whole by breaking down its internal and external factors that affect them daily. So it's not a one size fits all, since no two persons are the same. We're biologically different, and the factors that affect our experiences with health differ. Therefore, holistic nutrition looks at every aspect of our lives to uncover the root cause of a problem rather than just treating physical symptoms.

The practice of holistic nutrition began during the period of ancient civilization, particularly in Greece. Ancient Greeks believed that where we live, our income, education level, genetics, relationships with friends and family, and the condition of our environment can affect our health. Initially, doctors in this era understood diseases to be caused by an imbalance of the four bodily fluids, such as yellow bile, blood, black bile, and phlegm. External factors caused any imbalance. But if these fluids were balanced, it signified health. Other philosophers like Hippocrates further expanded on this idea about health.

Hippocrates was an ancient Greek physician who had a significant influence on the development of medicine. He believed that these four internal fluids would remain at equilibrium when we balance our lifestyle and environmental factors (such as water, food, and temperature). When this level of stability is established, we'll be healthier. But when one of these four fluids becomes dominant, we'll fall sick. So doctors practicing ancient Greek medicine treated patients by asking questions about the patient's lifestyle, diet, and other personal questions before administering suitable treatments. These old ideas about life and health laid the foundation for Western medicine to evolve into what it is today.

Today, wellness programs and educational approaches that emphasize the importance of a healthy diet and physical exercise can be traced back to the ancient Greeks, whose concepts and health knowledge focused on the whole person.

One of Hippocrates' famous quotes, "Let food be thy medicine," suggests that our diet can either make us sick or keep us healthy. So Hippocrates promoted the idea of eating a balanced diet and living a healthy lifestyle to treat and prevent diseases. So physicians practicing Hippocratic medicine treated illnesses and diseases using food and other natural remedies.

Hippocrates' understanding of food and health stemmed from the notion that different foods cause the body to produce different bodily fluids. Cold foods, for instance, produce phlegm in the body, while warm foods produce yellow bile. Ancient Greeks understood that different seasons affected the nature and balance of the four bodily fluids. Certain illnesses become dominant as the seasons change—likewise, the kinds of foods that were available. So doctors also used seasonal foods to treat diseases.

If a patient had chest problems, physicians would mix honey, vinegar, and barley soup together and give it to the patient to bring up phlegm. They also treated pain on the side of the ribs by applying a wet sponge to that area. Sometimes, a bath was given to a patient suffering from pneumonia to help raise the level of the phlegm.

Besides those treatments, there are other natural remedies that the ancient Greeks have gifted us with that we still use today to treat illnesses and diseases. They include:

- ***Using the oil from olives to include in sunscreen and treating skin problems like acne.*** Olives have been a staple in the Greek diet and medicine. It has been used for centuries as a folk remedy due to its anti-inflammatory and antimicrobial properties. Leaves of olive trees were ground to make a facial mask used to cure acne and other skin problems. Nowadays, people frequently use olive oil to treat damaged hair, help with minor cuts and bruises, and moisturize the skin.
- ***Horseradish to help with respiratory problems.*** People use this vegetable as a spice and condiment in their

meals worldwide. But in ancient times, it was eaten during the cold winter months to remove excess phlegm from parts of the respiratory system such as the lungs and sinuses. Today, horseradish is frequently used for sinus relief.

- **Beetroot to help with anemia.** The roots of the beet plant are very rich in iron, and we need iron in our bodies to make more red blood cells. So the ancient Greeks would make juice out of beetroots and offer them to patients suffering from anemia and other blood-related illnesses. Nowadays, most people use beetroots to prevent hair loss, treat dandruff, and brighten the skin.
- **Tomatoes to help prevent prostate cancer.** Tomatoes are very high in lycopene, a compound shown to reduce the risk of developing prostate cancer. Ancient Greeks believed that consuming at least one tomato a day would protect men against prostate cancer— most

certainly a tip worth noting if you're over the age of 40. Today, tomatoes are frequently used for skincare.

- *Using mint.* Ancient Greeks used mint to help relieve migraines and to relieve stomach aches. Mint is still used today to freshen breath and add flavour to water.
- *Consuming flaxseed to lower cholesterol.* Flaxseed is very high in healthy fat, fibre, and antioxidants. It's one of those superfoods that can boost your health when you eat it. Due to its nutritional value, it can help with digestion, lower cholesterol levels, and aid other health problems. So ancient physicians frequently prescribed it to treat illnesses. Today, people commonly use flaxseed to exfoliate and glow the skin and support hair growth.
- *Fennel for pain relief and weight loss.* Fennel is a layered, bulbous vegetable that resembles onions but isn't closely related to onions. It's frequently used in cooking to

enhance the flavour of the food. Every part of a fennel plant is edible, from the seeds to the bulb to the leaves. Ancient Greeks consumed fennel in the form of herbal tea to support weight loss, relieve menstrual cramps, and treat joint and muscle pain. Nowadays, fennel is commonly used to treat various digestive problems as well as relieve menstrual cramps.

There are many ancient Greek remedies, but these are only a few. These natural remedies are the foundation of holistic health today. Other ancient medical traditions based on holistic health include Ayurveda, traditional Chinese medicine, Western herbalism or traditional European medicine.

Why Is Holistic Nutrition So Important Today?

We need holistic health methods now more than ever because our healthcare system is failing us. Even using the word 'system,' which is supposed to mean a collection of professional care providers working together with individual patients to restore health, is an understatement for a service that can't care for us all. Our healthcare system cannot extend care to all those who need it. You may think that this problem stems from a shortage of hospitals, but that's not the case. Billions of dollars are allocated to the healthcare industry each year, so this problem isn't due to a shortage of hospitals. Instead, one of the problems is a shortage of staff.

Most hospitals don't have enough doctors. Globally, there aren't enough doctors to treat all patients needing medical care. In addition, the few physicians still in practice may choose to reduce their clinical hours due to burnout or other reasons. For a patient, this can mean you'll spend hours waiting in the emergency department for a doctor. The emergency department is a section of a hospital where people with life-threatening conditions go before the appropriate physician can attend to them. But people with non-life-threatening illnesses still go there. So what you have now is a place that's crowded with people waiting for hours for the limited number of doctors available. Waiting for hours can be very risky, especially if you have a critical condition that needs immediate help. I've heard of situations where people die in the emergency room as a result. So when there aren't enough doctors, there can be a delay in access to healthcare, which can be problematic.

This is one of the reasons why more and more people are beginning to demand natural alternatives to conventional medicine. Since doctors aren't available to save us all, the ball is in our court to protect ourselves. This is why we need to take a holistic approach to care by educating ourselves on how best to care for our health to keep illnesses at bay. In turn, it'll help us stay out of the emergency room.

Many of the diseases causing the most deaths worldwide are chronic illnesses. These are illnesses like asthma, diabetes, heart disease, and stroke that can last for a long time. Chronic diseases are preventable. Two of the leading causes of stroke and heart disease are high blood cholesterol and high blood pressure. High blood pressure is caused by eating too many salty foods. If the bulk of your diet comes from packaged, processed, and store-bought foods, you might be consuming more than the recommended daily amount of salt and predisposing yourself to stroke and heart disease. Thus, we should be consuming no more than five grams of salt a day. With junk foods, it's easy to consume more than recommended because of the high amounts of salt usually added to preserve and enhance their taste. So one way to reduce your salt intake is to eat healthy foods. Whole foods rich in potassium, such as fresh fruits and vegetables, lentils, nuts, beans, and starchy vegetables, can lower elevated blood pressure to a healthier range.

Eating foods high in saturated and trans fat can increase your blood cholesterol levels. When your blood cholesterol levels are high, you're at a higher risk of heart disease. Most saturated fats are found in animal products like dairy and high-fat meats, while trans fats are found in processed foods and junk foods. Both types of fat are harmful to the body in high amounts. So the best way to protect your health is to reduce your intake of saturated fats and eliminate sources of trans fat from your diet.

Even diabetes, particularly type-2 diabetes, is also caused by an unhealthy diet. This long-term condition is due to your body's inability to produce enough insulin—a hormone that's responsible for lowering your blood sugar level. The most significant risk factor for becoming diabetic is consuming too many sugary foods and calorie-dense foods, whether liquid or solid. Although these foods may look appealing, the more you consume them coupled with a sedentary lifestyle, the higher your chances of becoming overweight or obese. And being overweight or obese increases your likelihood of developing type-2 diabetes. So the best way to avoid type-2 diabetes is to feed your body with healthy foods. In addition, foods with high fibre content are excellent at preventing elevated blood sugar levels because they lower your blood sugar levels to a more beneficial range.

Moreover, the "Western" or "conventional" approach to health care is very different from alternative health services and approaches. The word "alternative" and "holistic" are sometimes used interchangeably to mean helping one deviate from conventional medicine. For example, when mainstream medicine doctors want to treat an illness, they typically administer pharmaceutical drugs, surgery, or radiation. But practitioners using alternative methods to help with practices like acupuncture, Reiki, massage therapy, meditation, chiropractic, herbal remedies, and nutritional therapies to stimulate our body's ability to help itself.

One of the problems with taking conventional treatments is that they frequently have side effects. No matter how minor these side effects are, they can still cause serious health problems. For example, a medicine to relieve aches and pain may cause nausea, rashes, or fever. Due to this problem, some people incorporate alternative treatments alongside their medications to help alleviate any side effects. Alternative or holistic therapies are generally safe non-invasive, and they serve as an additional option to managing illnesses and side effects of medications. They're excellent at helping with issues such as pain, poor sleep, anxiety, and so on. In addition, alternative methods could potentially help you reduce the use of certain medications. For example, acupuncture can help relieve pain caused by some chemotherapy drugs. You can likewise use acupuncture for stress management.

What's more, holistic health with nutrition can provide short and long-term benefits such as increased energy levels, stress management, a better quality of sleep, relief of headaches, etc., which can improve overall health. The focus of holistic nutrition is centred around using natural alternatives to better your well-being, so you'll be able to treat any ongoing problem. And in the long run, it'll protect you against illnesses.

Holistic medicines are intended to improve your health inside and outside. It includes using substances like antioxidant-rich foods and vitamins to enhance healing and prevent future illnesses. Due to its huge emphasis on prevention, holistic methods help avoid the need for repeated, costly treatments. I'm a huge proponent of holistic health because you can use it to help with a wide range of illnesses. It focuses on improving your overall well-being by rehibilitating your physical, mental, social, emotional, and spiritual health.

As you seek better ways of improving your health, you'll adopt new habits and lifestyle changes to enhance your well-being. This means you'll foster effective management techniques that will allow you to remain healthy in both the short-term and over the long haul. Knowledge of holistic methods gives you access to the tools and resources that will help you manage your condition more effectively.

The remaining chapters of this book will guide you through simple ways to help you with your health by using nutrition, natural supplementation, diet, and exercise. You will also read about how the five aspects of nutritional health will aid you in accomplishing your day-to-day activities with more energy and less stress on your body.

THE BENEFITS OF HOLISTIC NUTRITION

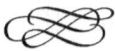

Moving toward a holistic approach with nutrition teaches you how to eat. It's not a diet; it's a way of life. It empowers you to make the right food choices without feeling guilty. What we eat doesn't just affect our physical health. It affects other aspects of our well-being. We can only eat a certain amount of food on any given day. Since the bulk of the nutrients come from these foods, it's wise to choose foods that not only meet your caloric needs but are rich in nutrients.

You can begin to eat nutrient-rich foods by incorporating more natural, plant-based foods into your diet and avoiding junk and processed foods. The key to eating well is to make sure you're consuming a balanced diet with lots of vegetables on your plate. Eating healthy foods provides you with a lifetime of healthy living and longevity. They also make you feel better overall. It becomes a lifestyle as you stick to eating healthy foods over time.

When we eat is also an essential part of healthy eating. Nutrition experts recommend we eat three meals a day to give our bodies time to digest the food and use the nutrients, implying that we should eat breakfast, lunch, and dinner daily. Skipping a meal or waiting too long to eat may jeopardize your healthy lifestyle. In addition, you may be tempted to eat unhealthy foods or overeat during any one meal.

How Can Holistic Nutrition Help You?

Eating nutrient-rich foods can have several positive effects on your body, such as:

- **Weight loss**: There's no magic to weight loss. It's all about calories in vs. calories out. You need to be in a caloric deficit to lose weight, which implies you need to consume fewer calories than you burn. If, for instance, your body burns 2,000 calories a day to provide energy to fuel your cells and organs, consuming less than 2,000 calories will result in weight loss. The healthier way to lose weight is to focus on losing one to two pounds of weight a week. Anything past that may lead to other health problems.

Many people turn to fad diets and supplements promising immediate results to lose weight. While it's possible to shed pounds in a short time, it isn't healthy for you. A safer and more sustainable way to lose weight is to make dietary and lifestyle changes. This means cutting off all unhealthy foods and replacing them with healthier ones.

Processed/junk foods tend to be higher in calories than natural, unprocessed foods mainly because they contain higher amounts of sugar and fat, increasing their caloric content. So the easiest way to ensure you're eating fewer calories than you burn is to eat foods that keep you satiated for more extended periods to prevent cravings. This includes whole foods like potatoes, nuts and seeds, fruits and vegetables, whole grains, legumes, and lean meat and fish.

Whole foods are also rich in fibre. Dietary fibre helps to fill the stomach and make you feel less hungry. But junk/processed foods do the opposite. They're low in dietary fibre. As such, they elevate your blood glucose. When your blood glucose is high, your brain sends out hormonal signals encouraging you to eat more. So over time, you can become obese or diabetic from prolonged elevated blood glucose. However, whole foods are very effective at controlling the release of glucose into the blood. So when you eat fibre-rich foods, they help release glucose slowly into the blood. This helps maintain your blood glucose level, sustain energy, control your appetite, and prevent overeating.

- **Helps with digestion and bloating:** Bloating occurs when you retain gas in your digestive tract (aka gastrointestinal tract or GI tract), specifically in the large intestine. The large intestine contains good bacteria that help break down foods or parts of food that aren't completely digested. These harmless bacteria digest foods through a process called fermentation and produce gas as a waste product. When gas accumulates, your abdomen may feel full and painful or become swollen. Bloating is typically accompanied by frequent belching, rumbling in the gut, and excessive farting. Anyone can experience bloating. Bloating can also be caused by swallowing air while you eat, the type of food you eat, or medical conditions like GI disorders.

Some foods can make you bloated. Foods like dairy, excessive fibre, artificial sweeteners, sugar alcohols, fructose, gluten, junk foods, among others, can cause bloating. Since junk/processed foods are very high in sugar and fat and low in fibre, they can also cause bloating. Fat takes longer to digest than protein and carbohydrates. So when you eat high-fat foods like ice cream or pastries, it keeps the stomach feeling full longer. In some people, this may result in bloating. And since unhealthy foods are very low in fibre, you may not be stooling regularly, making you more bloated. Dietary fibre helps increase bowel movement and decrease the duration of time your stool stays in your colon. The longer your stool stays stuck in your colon, the more time those good bacteria have to break them down through the process of fermentation and produce gas.

The sensible strategy to get rid of bloating is to adjust your diet. You can start by incorporating varieties of whole foods into your diet. Since whole foods are rich in fibre, you should increase their intake gradually to give your colon enough time to adapt to this dietary change to minimize gas and bloating. It sounds counterproductive that the same dietary fibre that helps reduce bloating can also cause bloating if consumed excessively, but you must make a gradual dietary change to avoid it.

How much fibre is enough? For a healthy diet, dieticians recommend adults increase their average daily fibre intake to 10 grams by eating five servings of vegetables, two servings of fruits, and about five servings of cereals and grains daily.

- **Alleviates stress and anxiety:** Stress is inevitable. We all experience stress from our relationships, jobs, or regular day-to-day activities.

But not all stress is bad. Sometimes, we need a little bit of stress to push us to accomplish something and to adapt to new situations. However, stress becomes harmful to our bodies when it's prolonged. For example, if you consistently overwork yourself with barely enough sleep, you're experiencing stress. In addition, chronic stress can lead to other health problems if this behaviour persists for months.

When you're under stress, your body releases stress hormones like cortisol, epinephrine, and norepinephrine into the blood. At the same time, your body undergoes physiological changes like increased heart rate and blood pressure. Your immune cells also become activated and released into the blood, where they'll migrate to tissues that are more likely to be damaged from physical force (e.g., the skin). During stress, your body begins to break down your energy reserves and direct this energy to tissues and organs that need it the most, like the brain and skeletal muscle. At the same time, crucial processes like reproduction, digestion, and the production of growth hormones will shut down.

But when the stress is frequent or chronic, a sustained increase in blood pressure will cause your heart to work harder. As a result, your immunity will become suppressed, and your immune cells won't be able to protect you against illnesses. Even anxiety can add more stress to your body. The feeling of worry, unease, or fear can cause a similar stress response.

One of the problems with chronic stress is that it uses up the body's nutrient stores, so you may feel tired and lack energy during these times. This is because stress uses many nutrients to produce energy, even if we're sedentary all day. This happens because your body is trying to maintain balance, so it uses a more significant amount of specific nutrients in the process. As a result, nutrients like vitamin C, B-vitamins, iron, magnesium, zinc, and vitamin D may end up depleted during stress.

If your diet doesn't supply all the nutrients your body needs, it can exacerbate your stress response and cause an imbalance in your stress hormones. For example, when you're feeling stressed, you may have noticed your hunger levels increase, and the desire for fatty, sugary, and processed foods, may increase. We feel this way because the hormone cortisol makes us crave these foods.

To help replenish any lost nutrients, focus on eating a balanced diet to help provide these nutrients. With a healthy diet, you can reduce stress and eliminate stress-related illnesses. Adopting a diet high in fruits and vegetables, legumes, whole grains, monounsaturated fat, omega-3 fatty acids, nuts and seeds, eggs, and lean meat, can have antioxidative and anti-inflammatory properties against stress.

Supplementation with vitamins and minerals can equally reduce stress. Taking supplements can help provide the body with nutrients absent from the diet or not provided in the required amount. So supplementing your diet with manganese, calcium, vitamin C and E, magnesium, B vitamins can protect the body against stress.

- **Relieves headaches:** Headache is a frequent illness that people of all ages experience. It's a pain that can happen at one or both sides of your head, all over your head, or at the sinus regions on your face. And this pain can sometimes be severe or mild and last for either a short or long time.

DIFFERENT THINGS CAN CAUSE HEADACHES, like inadequate sleep, side effects of medications, dehydration, stress, diet, and other underlying health problems. Numerous studies have shown that foods that contain large amounts of substances like nitrites, biogenic amines (e.g., phenylethylamine, histamine, and tyramine), monosodium glutamate (MSG), artificial sweeteners, and gluten can trigger headaches. You can easily find these substances in processed foods by reading the ingredients listed under the nutritional facts label.

MSG, for instance, is a flavour enhancer used in various packaged foods, sauces, and soups. Manufacturers may sometimes use other names like hydrolyzed plant protein, kombu extract, natural flavour, flavouring, and hydrolyzed vegetable protein to suggest its addition.

Headache can be triggered by excessive caffeine use, alcoholic beverages, and chocolate (which contains a tyramine-like substance called phenylethylamine). So one of the best ways to relieve headaches is to cut off processed foods from your diet and incorporate more whole foods.

Numerous researchers indicate that magnesium-rich foods may help relieve headaches by relaxing the blood vessels carrying blood to the head. High amounts of magnesium can be found in foods like avocado, dark leafy greens, and tuna. Likewise, increasing your intake of healthy fats such as omega-3 fatty acids may also relieve headaches. Foods rich in omega-3 fatty acids include legumes, salmon, seeds, and mackerel.

Fruits, particularly those with high water content, are good for headaches. If a headache is caused by dehydration, then rehydrating yourself is all that's needed. You can also drink water to relieve a headache.

Even the antioxidants found in fruits and vegetables can help with headaches. During the digestion of food, our bodies produce free radicals as waste products. However, when we consume high amounts of processed foods, our bodies produce excessive amounts of free radicals, which can cause oxidative stress in the body. And this can trigger a headache. So consuming foods rich in antioxidants can help stop oxidative stress as well as headaches.

If a headache is caused by low blood sugar, consuming more whole grains, legumes, and healthy fat can help to increase glycogen stores in the brain and maintain your blood glucose.

- **Improves the look of the skin:** It's well known that what we eat affects the appearance of our skin. The skin is the largest organ in the body. It's made up of fats, minerals, water, and protein. The skin helps to protect us against germs and regulates our body temperature. Our lifestyle, the genes we inherit, and other internal and external factors can affect how our skin looks.

In terms of diet, poor eating habits and imbalance in nutrition can age our skin and make it look dull. A diet high in sugar can cause premature ageing and increase the appearance of wrinkles on the skin. When you consume sugary foods, the excess sugar circulating in the blood can bind to the protein and fat molecules on the skin. Protein molecules such as collagen and elastin located on the skin help support the skin's structure. Collagen prevents our skin from sagging by giving us a plump, youthful look. At the same time, elastin keeps our skin flexible. So too much sugar in the blood can bind to the collagen molecules and damage them.

By consuming a healthy and balanced diet, you can improve the look of the skin. Foods high in dietary fibre, such as whole foods, are excellent at preventing elevated blood glucose. More So foods rich in antioxidants (vitamins A, C, and E) have anti-ageing effects on the skin. Vitamin E is the primary antioxidant required by the skin. Our body doesn't have stores for vitamin E, so we must continually consume foods rich in vitamin E to get this nutrient. Some good sources of vitamin E include vegetables, fruits, nuts and seeds, plant-based oils, some meats, and dairy products.

Vitamin C is the second antioxidant required for healthier-looking skin. This nutrient helps to stabilize the collagen on our skin. Just like vitamin E, our body doesn't produce or store vitamin C, so eating citrus fruits and vegetables is the best method of restoring our body's reserves. Vitamin A is another nutrient that can function in an antioxidant role in the body. It can be found in foods such as yellow, orange, and red coloured fruits and vegetables, mango, cantaloupe, watermelon, strawberries, tomatoes, carrots, and sweet potatoes.

Besides vitamins and minerals, our skin requires enough water to function properly, just like our body. Health experts recommend drinking at least two litres of water a day for optimal health. Insufficient water intake can cause the skin on our lips and other parts of our body to appear dull. Other trace nutrients like copper, zinc, iodine and iron are equally vital for improving the appearance of our skin.

While fats are often perceived as something unhealthy, they are indeed one of the main components of skin health. So which fats should we be consuming? Both omega-3 and omega-6 fatty acids. Omega-3 fatty acids can be found in salmon, sardines, walnuts, chia seeds, and hemp seeds. While sources of omega-6 include nuts and seeds, soybeans, meat, fish, eggs, and poultry. These healthy fats help form our skin's structure, prevent moisture loss, and maintain plump and glowing skin.

- **Stabilizes your mood:** Mood is a positive or negative emotional state that can last for a long or short time. Your mood can be affected by your lifestyle, such as diet and other internal and external factors. When it comes to diet, some foods, especially foods with low nutritional value, may leave us feeling drained after consuming them. Foods like processed snacks and sugar-sweetened beverages are the biggest culprit.

The connection between our diet and mood stems from our gut and brain's chemical and physical connection. When we consume healthy foods, the "good" bacteria in our gut produce chemicals called neurotransmitters sent to the brain, positively affecting our mood. But a steady intake of junk food causes inflammation in the body, which hinders the communication between your gut and your brain.

So the best way to reduce mood fluctuations is to stick to a healthy diet consisting of whole, unprocessed foods with sufficient protein, healthy fats, and dietary fibre. For instance, consuming, complex carbohydrates like whole grains and legumes can signal our brains to release the feel-good hormone serotonin. Serotonin is a natural mood stabilizer. Normal levels of this hormone in the brain will leave you feeling happier, less anxious, more emotionally stable, and calmer.

Likewise, foods rich in antioxidants, vitamins, and minerals such as fruits and vegetables may help to stabilize our mood.

Antioxidants prevent oxidative stress to brain cells that can cause mood disorders like anxiety and depression. In turn, we'll feel less depressed and happier.

- **Balances your hormones:** Your body uses the nutrients supplied from your diet to regulate your hormones. For instance, the steroid hormones—testosterone, progesterone, and estrogen—require cholesterol to be synthesized. These hormones are among the most critical hormones in the body. They regulate many body systems and processes essential for our survival.

Several factors can cause your hormones to fluctuate. One of such factors is consuming a poor diet. Digestive problems and inflammation related to a poor diet can cause hormonal imbalance. When our hormones fluctuate, we may experience trouble sleeping, irritability, weight gain, and fatigue. So how can we balance our hormones? By consuming a nutritious diet filled with unprocessed whole foods from diverse food groups, we can get all the essential macronutrients and micronutrients necessary to balance our hormones.

Magnesium is perhaps one of the most fundamental nutrients to help balance hormones. It regulates the stress hormone cortisol. Cortisol controls other processes within the body, such as your immune response and metabolism. Certain foods such as processed and junk foods may cause inflammation in the body that can elevate your cortisol levels. However, a sufficient intake of magnesium may help calm down elevated cortisol levels by inhibiting the activation of the adrenal gland that releases this hormone. So to ensure you're getting enough magnesium from your diet, consume more dark leafy greens, pumpkin seeds, chia seeds, chickpeas, lentils, black beans, and avocado.

Other hormones like thyroid hormone may fluctuate if your diet isn't providing trace nutrients like iodine, selenium, and iron. These nutrients are essential for the production of thyroid hormones. One of the thyroid hormone functions is to regulate your metabolic rate—the rate at which you gain and lose weight. A diet that's lacking in these nutrients may cause your thyroid levels to become low, a condition known as hypothyroidism. When this occurs, your metabolism will slow down, and you may gain weight. So if you're trying to manage your weight, incorporate foods such as seaweeds, whole grains, leafy vegetables, dairy products, fish, meat, legumes, and poultry, which are rich in these nutrients, into your diet.

Your overall nutrition can affect the circulating levels of certain hormones like ghrelin. Ghrelin is a hormone that regulates our appetite. When we're hungry, our body releases large amounts of ghrelin into the bloodstream, which increases the feeling of hunger. But during periods of satiety and fullness, our ghrelin levels are low. Numerous studies have shown that high levels of ghrelin in the body can increase our desire for high-fat and carbohydrate-dense meals and cause us to overeat.

So how can we regulate the hunger hormone? First, consuming a healthy diet consisting of whole grains can keep you feeling full longer due to their high fibre content, which may help balance the hunger hormone and prevent overeating. What's more, combining healthy fats with fibre-rich foods can increase the satiating potential of fat and reduce your food intake.

Ensuring your diet provides sufficient B-vitamins is also an excellent idea when your hormones fluctuate. B-vitamins can be found in animal protein sources.

- **You'll have more energy:** Any food you eat that has calories will give you energy, but not all foods affect your energy levels the same. Some foods cause an immediate boost in energy, which is usually followed by a rapid decline. While other foods keep your energy levels up for a long time. So what you eat can either keep you energized or make you feel sluggish.

Of all the three macronutrients, carbohydrates are the quickest to digest, and fats are the slowest. Carbs are your body's preferred energy source. So the composition of your diet can affect your energy levels. There are different types of carbohydrates with varying effects on how much energy you have. Simple carbs have either one or two sugar molecules, known as monosaccharides and disaccharides. Because of their simple structure, our body can quickly digest them to provide energy. Examples include fruit juices, white bread, processed products with added sugars, and candy.

Simple carbs are usually low in fibre, so they have a high glycemic index. Implying that they'll cause your blood sugar levels to rise and fall rapidly, which can leave you feeling tired after eating. This is why you feel sleepy and tired after consuming sugary and processed foods.

On the other hand, complex carbs have three or more sugar molecules known as polysaccharides and oligosaccharides, so they take longer to digest. Complex carbs are usually high in fibre and have a low glycemic index. Implying that they gradually increase your blood sugar levels. Some examples of complex carbs include whole, unprocessed grains, legumes, fruits, vegetables, and starches.

So if you want to feel energized throughout the day, eat a balanced diet that's rich in complex carbs, protein, fruits, vegetables, and "small amounts" of healthy fats. Proteins help slow down the rate at which your body absorbs the carbs. And yes, I emphasized small amounts of fats because foods high in fat can stimulate your brain to produce serotonin, making you feel tired and sluggish.

- **You'll understand your body better:** As phenotypically and genetically different as we all are, so do our needs differ. Our bodies require different things depending on our goals. If your goal is to maintain weight, your food intake quantity, composition, and timing might differ from someone trying to lose weight.

It can take some time to figure out what works for you and what doesn't since there are various ways of eating healthier. And healthy eating is different for everybody depending on your lifestyle and other underlying factors. But a careful examination of your food choices and how your body responds to them can help you understand your body better. It takes a lot of observations and practice to find what works for you.

The more you pay attention to your body, you may notice patterns in the way certain foods make you feel or if you need to stock up on certain nutrients. Listening and eating mindfully can help you form a healthier relationship with food. By eating mindfully, you'll become aware of those subtle bodily sensations, food triggers, and emotions, which can help you discover how different foods impact your everyday life, mind, and body.

You might realize that certain foods make you sluggish in the morning, while others energize you and improve your focus and attention. Or you might discover that you only eat a particular food when you're sad. The goal of understanding how your body responds to your diet is to be able to take actions that better support your body's needs.

NUTRITION CONCEPTS AND GUT HEALTH

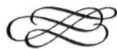

Hippocrates once claimed, "All disease begins in the gut." As cliche as it sounds, he was correct with his assumption. The gut is like a powerhouse within our body. It breaks down what we eat to provide nutrients and energy to function daily. It also affects our immune system and communicates with our brain through the vagus nerve and hormones, which helps to maintain our overall health. Our gut can perform these functions through the help of the billions of microorganisms that reside in it.

There are numerous microorganisms all over our bodies, both inside and outside.

They're so small that we can't see them through our naked eyes, but they're essential to our health. Each microbe performs a different function in our body. The collection of all the microbes in and on our body is known as the human microbiome. The human microbiome comprises bacteria, viruses, archaea, and eukaryotic microbes all living together. These organisms aren't just restricted to one location in the body. Each part of the body has a specific amount of microbial community it can contain. Generally, if a body part/structure has a large surface area, it'll contain much more microbe than a body part with a smaller surface area, which is the case with the intestines.

The intestines are an essential structure in our gut. The intestine walls are covered in folds, and if you were to flatten out the entire intestine wall, it would be about the size of a tennis court! This is because so many microbes cover the entire walls of the intestines, creating a very dense microbial community. Thus, we can say that the gut contains the largest, densest, and most diverse microbial community in our body. Although different microbes coexist together in the gut, bacteria are the predominant microorganisms you'll find from the mouth to the intestines. The microbial community located in our gut is called the gut microbiome.

The gut microbiome is essential because these diverse and complex microbial communities help us carry out many chemical reactions and break down substances that we cannot digest on our own. There are "good" and "bad" bacteria in our gut. Anything we eat either causes our body to produce more of the good or bad bacteria. The good bacteria do more than help us digest our food. They prevent the bad bacteria from increasing in quantity. If there are more bad bacteria than good, you'll become sick and vice versa. When the good bacteria decreases, you may begin to experience gastrointestinal problems like diarrhea, abdominal pain, bloating, constipation, vomiting, and heartburn. Some diseases like diabetes, inflammatory bowel disease, and cancer, among others, have also been linked to changes in gut microbial composition.

Why is gut health so important? Our gut can affect our overall health. It can affect our digestion, our mood, our immune system, and the health of our brain. Since the vagus nerve physically connects our gut to our brain, anything the gut secretes affects the brain, and the brain can release chemicals that also affect our gut. For example, our gut produces short-chain fatty acids (SCFA) compounds after digesting fibre-rich food. SCFA can leave the gut and go to the brain region that controls our appetite to reduce our food intake.

Likewise, our gut releases chemicals called neurotransmitters that can affect the brain regions that control our feelings and emotions. Just like our brain, our gut produces neurotransmitters such as serotonin and gamma-aminobutyric acid (GABA). Serotonin is the feel-good hormone. It's a chemical that affects our brain to make us feel happy, while GABA controls our feelings of fear and anxiety.

Our gut equally affects our immune system. The gut and the brain are connected through the immune system. If our immune system is activated for too long, it can lead to inflammation associated with brain disorders like Alzheimer's disease, dementia, and depression. An unhealthy gut can produce inflammatory toxins that can leak into the blood and activate your immune system. If your gut keeps producing inflammatory toxins, it can lead to brain disorders. So you can improve the health of your brain and your immune system by keeping your gut healthy.

What Are the Best Foods to Eat?

Overeating junk food can affect the composition of your gut microbiome and cause more harmful bacteria to become dominant. So the best foods to eat consist of whole foods, fish, and lean meat. Consuming a healthy diet helps you maintain a healthy microbial balance.

When it comes to gut health, how these healthy foods are combined is very important. Some food combinations can leave us feeling bloated and cause other gut problems, while others seem to help us maintain a flat belly. This is because certain foods pair well while others don't. Before providing you with examples of foods to combine, let's first understand the concept of food combining. Food combining is the process of pairing different types of foods together in a meal in such a way that they help your gut function better. The idea behind food combining is to only pair foods that support good health and digestion. No one wants to deal with a grumbling stomach all day or a distended abdomen filled with gas while out with friends. So the composition of your diet can either make or break a good day. With proper food combining, you can significantly improve the digestion and absorption of certain foods.

The rules for properly pairing foods are as follows:

- *Don't combine starchy food with acidic food.* Starchy foods like potato, bread, and grains are digested by enzymes that work best when the gut is less acidic and more alkaline. While acidic foods, which are your protein sources (e.g., meat, legumes, fish, etc.), are digested by enzymes that thrive in acidic pH. Proponents of food-combining diets believe we should separate these two food groups because our bodies may not digest them simultaneously. It's like asking our digestive systems to be alkaline and acidic at the same time. Instead,

combine non-starchy foods (e.g., brussels sprouts, asparagus, celery, carrots, cauliflower, onions, cabbage, and broccoli) with any protein source of your choice.
- ***Fruits should only be eaten on an empty stomach, particularly melons.*** Fruits digest very fast, so eating them on an empty stomach can help to replenish fluids, vitamins, and minerals quickly. Melons (e.g., watermelon) have a very high water content, so eating it together with a solid food can dilute the pH of your gut and make it more alkaline. That's a problem for the enzyme *pepsin*, which digests protein only when the gut is acidic. If this happens, digestion can be delayed until the acidic environment of your gut is restored.
- ***Eat fruits and vegetables separately.*** Fruits and vegetables are very different foods that digest differently. Various fruits and vegetables contain digestive enzymes that might speed up the

digestive process. But fruits have more sugar, and some food-combining purists believe excess sugar can delay the digestion of vegetables.

- ***Don't combine different sources of protein together.*** The idea that plant protein sources contain incomplete amino acids and that we need to combine different plant protein sources to form a complete protein became popular in the 1970s. But this has since been discredited by the medical community. If you consume diverse plant protein sources throughout the day, it can supply all the required amino acids your body needs. However, amino acid deficiency can become a problem when your diet isn't diverse in plant protein sources but consists of large quantities of one type of plant protein.
- ***Dairy products should only be eaten on an empty stomach, particularly milk.*** Dairy products are rich in protein and calcium. Our body

needs protein for muscle growth and repair, while calcium is required to build and maintain strong bones and teeth. Some dairy products are solid (e.g., cheese), while others are liquid (e.g., milk). Compared to solids, liquids digest quicker. So if you drink milk on an empty stomach, your body will readily absorb all the nutrients in it. Milk is a good source of magnesium and phosphorus, and some are fortified with vitamin D. These nutrients help our body absorb and use the calcium in milk.

Alkalize the Body

Different foods have different effects on the pH of your body. Theories about how certain foods keep us healthy because they balance our blood pH, while certain foods lead to diseases because they lower the blood's pH began in the 20th century. pH is a measure of how acidic or alkaline a solution is. It's typically measured on a scale of 1 to 14, with 7 being neutral. So if the pH of the solution is less than 7, the solution is acidic. But if the pH is greater than 7, the solution is alkaline.

Our blood has a pH within the range of 7.35 to 7.45. The pH of our blood differs from that of other fluids in our body. This is the alkaline level at which cells and organs can function optimally. But when it drops below 7.35, our blood becomes acidic, which is dangerous for our health. Anything greater than the pH of 7.45 is an alkaline environment that's harmful to us. It's quite difficult for the pH of our blood to fall off this optimal range because our body has effective strategies to regulate its pH balance. However, our diet can cause tiny fluctuations within the normal range.

Our bodies have several ways to regulate the pH of the blood:

- Through the bicarbonate buffering system that's present in our blood.
- By releasing carbon dioxide from our blood when we exhale.
- By removing hydrogen ions from the blood through our urine.

These natural mechanisms help our body maintain a healthy pH range.

Every food item has its own pH value. Lime, for instance, has a pH less than four, while tofu has a pH of 7.2. When we consume these foods, they get broken down, and by-products or metabolic wastes are generated. This waste product is believed to alter our body's pH. It can have an alkaline, acidic, or neutral effect on the body, depending on what was consumed. In other words, if you eat foods that generate acidic waste products, your blood may become acidic.

We can group the foods we eat into acidic, alkaline, and neutral:

- **Acidic:** dairy, poultry, meat, grains, alcohol, fish, and eggs
- **Alkaline:** legumes, nuts, vegetables, and fruits
- **Neutral:** starches, healthy fats, and sugars

Acidic foods produce acidic waste products like sulphur and phosphate, while alkaline foods leave alkaline by-products such as calcium, potassium, and magnesium.

The idea of eating alkaline foods and following an alkaline diet has become widespread among celebrities. Alkaline foods can balance and maintain our blood pH. Regulating our blood pH can help maintain a constant internal environment for our cells and keep us healthy. However, when large amounts of acidic wastes are produced, the pH buffering systems in our body may not balance our pH, leading to diseases effectively.

Besides eating acidic foods, acidic by-products in our blood can come from the breakdown of glucose and glycogen without oxygen. When these compounds are broken down, lactic acid is generated. Lactic acid generates the proton that lowers the pH of our blood. It's generally produced in our skeletal muscles and our adipose tissue. When there is poor oxygen supply in the body, more lactic acid will be produced. Our pH levels can also decrease when our body generates ketone bodies during the breakdown of fat stored in our liver.

Together, all these processes, plus not eating enough fruits and vegetables, can further decrease the pH of your blood, which is deadly for your cells. Chronic low blood pH can damage your kidneys, cause your muscles to waste away, generate inflammation, or lead to osteoporosis. However, several studies conducted on humans have noted that eating fruits and vegetables can improve the pH of our blood to a normal range. In addition, the alkalizing waste products generated after consuming these foods can help you neutralize any excess acid in your blood and eliminate acid build-up. So consuming more whole, unprocessed foods and fruits and vegetables can alkalize your body.

One way to monitor your body's internal state is to monitor the pH of your urine. If it has a pH over 7, that tells you that your cells and organs are in an alkaline environment. A urine pH less than 7 tells you the opposite.

Eliminate Toxins

The amount of toxins we encounter daily is staggering. In our bodies, toxins are those normal waste products from the breakdown of food and respiration. Our bodies naturally eliminate toxins in our stool, urine, and sweat.

We don't need any special diet to eliminate toxins. The liver, skin, lungs, colon, and kidneys are our body's natural detoxifying systems.

The liver regulates many functions in our bodies. For example, it converts the nutrients from the foods we eat into substances our bodies can use, stores them, and releases them when needed. It also converts toxic substances into harmless products that our bodies can use or eliminate. After digestion, the blood carrying both nutrients and waste or toxic substances flows to the liver before moving to other parts of the body. Once in the liver, the blood is filtered, and any substance in the blood is either detoxified, removed from the blood, altered, or passed back to the blood.

The lungs are equally good at getting rid of substances that don't belong in them. They expel waste in the form of carbon dioxide gas from our bodies when we exhale. They also have tiny fibres called cilia that push contaminants out. So, if you inhale any toxic substance, they get trapped by the cilia, and you'll be able to cough it up.

The colon, also known as the large intestine, also eliminates toxins from our bodies.

The membrane that lines our intestines helps our bodies absorb nutrients and reject toxins and waste. After the small intestines have absorbed all nutrients from food, the undigested remains and rejected substances are passed to the colon to be eliminated into the feces.

Likewise, your kidneys are there to filter out all the waste products from digestion and other unwanted materials from your blood and flush them out of your body in your urine.

Your skin protects you against environmental toxins. But it's also an elimination route. For example, when you sweat, if there are too many water-soluble harmful substances in your blood, your body can flush them out. The oil on our skin can also eliminate fat-soluble toxins. Typically, our liver will convert fat-soluble toxins to water-soluble toxins; then, the kidneys will flush them out. But if the liver/kidneys are congested with toxins, the body will force them out through the skin. So the pimples, blackheads, and acne on your skin may be because of that.

Because our bodies naturally detoxify

themselves, toxins won't build up in a way our bodies can't excrete them. However, waste and harmful substances can accumulate in our blood and cause diseases if the body's detoxifying systems aren't healthy. When too much waste and toxins accumulate in the body, it can damage enzymes and make them not function properly. Enzymes help to speed up chemical reactions in the body. So a damaged enzyme implies those bodily processes will occur at a much slower pace, and your body won't function properly as a result. Our bodies rely on enzymes for every biological process.

What's more, accumulated toxins can damage those organs that help your body detoxify, making it harder for your body to eliminate toxins, which can create other health problems.

Some toxins damage the surface of cells. Cells communicate with themselves by sending signals to the proteins attached to the surface of another cell. Damage to this cell layer prevents it from getting information from other cells to respond properly.

That said, consuming certain foods can enhance our body's natural detoxification system and help to eliminate toxins. For example, foods like asparagus, spinach, kale, beets, avocado, grapefruit, and collard greens are rich in vitamins and antioxidants. As a result, they can assist our body's natural ability to cleanse and detoxify itself.

How Do Certain Foods Impact Our Bodies?

Each component of a healthy diet supplies our body with a different type of nutrient that influences our health. When you change your diet to a much healthier one, you'll get a deeper understanding of how these foods impact your health. A balanced diet is made up of the following:

- **Fruits and vegetables:** All foods have some vitamins and minerals, but fruits and vegetables are very high in specific vitamins and minerals such as antioxidants (e.g., vitamin A, C, E, and selenium), folic acid (aka vitamin B-9), vitamins B-6 and B-12. Vitamins and minerals are essential to our body because they perform diverse roles beneficial to our health.

For example, Vitamin A helps protect our body against oxidative stress, boosts our immunity to protect us against diseases, and maintains the tissue in our skin, respiratory, and digestive tract healthy. Examples of foods rich in Vitamin A include leafy greens, carrots, sweet potatoes, and watercress.

Vitamin C equally boosts our immunity and protects our body against oxidative stress. It also helps our body absorb iron from the foods we eat. In addition, it speeds up wound healing and keeps our gums healthy. Sources of vitamin C include strawberries, currants, green leafy vegetables, mangoes, avocados, and kiwi.

The B-vitamins, particularly B-9, B-6, and B-12, protect our hearts against diseases. In addition, they help our immune system function better and strengthen the connection and interaction between our brain and spinal cord. These vitamins also help our bodies break down proteins and manufacture proteins. You can find these vitamins in whole grains, dark leafy greens, nuts, seeds, legumes, and animal protein sources.

Fruits and vegetables also provide fibre and phytonutrients to our bodies. Phytonutrients are those compounds found in fruits and vegetables that have anti-inflammatory properties. They are equally excellent at enhancing our immunity, protecting against cancer, and helping to eliminate toxins from the body. The colour of a fruit or vegetable tells you what phytonutrient it has. So by eating diverse colours of fruits and vegetables, you'll be getting a variety of beneficial phytonutrients into your body.

There are seven phytonutrients found in fruits and vegetables. They include:

- Indole-3-carbinol: found in Brussel sprouts, cabbage, kale, broccoli, and turnips.
- Quercetin: found in garlic and onions.
- Lutein: found in kale, Swiss chard, and parsley.
- Anthocyanins: found in apples, blueberries, cherries, raspberries, and grapes.

- Limonene: found in limes, oranges, lemons, and tangerines.
- Carotenoids: found in apricots, squash, pumpkin, carrots, and peaches.
- Lycopene: found in red pepper, watermelon, tomatoes, and radishes.
- Whole grains: Whole grains offer numerous health benefits. The fibre in them makes them excellent at controlling our appetite and keeping us full for long. Dietary fibre also helps to prevent our blood sugar levels from spiking.

Moreover, because they're natural and unprocessed, they support the growth of good bacteria in the gut. Whole grains are known to cause our gut to release the feel-good hormone serotonin to regulate our mood and sleep.

The fibre in them equally helps to remove toxins from our body by binding to the toxic substances in our gut to ensure they're eliminated in our feces.

Sources of whole grains that you can

incorporate into your diet include brown rice, oats, quinoa, millet, barley, and cornmeal.

- **Proteins:** There are plant and animal sources of protein. If you eat meat, stay away from the processed ones, and opt for the leanest cuts because they're low in saturated fat. Likewise, choose grass-fed meats over corn-fed meats because they're more anti-inflammatory. Dairy products are also good protein sources, but they can be high in saturated fat. Choose skim or low-fat versions for a healthier alternative. Or, if you want to reduce your saturated fat intake drastically, include more plant protein sources in your diet.

Our bodies need protein for a lot of things. Protein keeps us feeling full longer. Our bodies use protein to build our muscles and make connective tissues for our bones, skin, and cartilage. Moreover, proteins regulate our blood sugar level and prevent spikes in blood sugar. It equally helps our adrenal and thyroid glands to function better.

Protein sources include nuts and seeds, whole grains, fish, meat, poultry, milk, lentils, legumes, peanuts, nut-butters, soy, and eggs.

- **Fats and oils:** We need some fat in our diet to be healthy. Fats can be found in animal protein sources and some plants. Eating healthy fats such as omega-3 fatty acids and plant sources of fat are more beneficial to our health. As much as possible, minimize your intake of animal fats.

Small amounts of fat in our diet help us absorb fat-soluble vitamins. They also insulate our organs. Fats are essential components of our cell membranes. Moreover, oils from plants, nuts, seeds, and omega-3 fatty acids decrease inflammation in our bodies. Fats equally lubricate our skin and keep our joints healthy. Likewise, our bodies use fat to make hormones.

Good fat sources include chia seeds, tuna, salmon, mackerel, almonds, walnuts, omega-3 enriched eggs, tofu, soybeans, flaxseed, and dark green vegetables.

Plant oils such as grapeseed oil, cocoa butter, avocado oil, corn oil, and coconut oil are also beneficial to our bodies.

THE BODY SYSTEMS

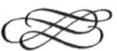

Our bodies are made up of complex internal structures and systems that influence one another and carry out critical biological processes from head to toe. Each body system is comprised of different structures that work together to serve a common purpose. Think of a body system as a house. Your house can't function as a place of safety if there aren't any doors installed. Likewise, you can't fully enjoy living in such a house if it isn't furnished. We can say the same for all the organ systems in our bodies. Each part of a system depends on other components to accomplish tasks that a single part can't do.

There are numerous organ systems inside

our body that manage essential body functions. Each body system also communicates and works with other organ systems to keep us alive and maintain our health. For example, the nutrients absorbed by the gut (digestive system) are carried to other body parts through the blood (circulatory system).

Our body systems rely on a healthy diet to supply all the essential nutrients required to function. The proteins, vitamins, minerals, healthy fats, and carbohydrates are what our organ systems use as building blocks to provide energy and nourish us. So with proper nutrition, your body can work at its full potential to keep you healthy.

SYSTEMS of the Body and Nutrition

Let's go over a few organ systems and how each plays a role in our overall holistic health.

- **Digestive system**

The digestive system comprises the gastrointestinal tract (GI tract or gut) and other organs that secrete substances to facilitate the digestive process, such as the liver, gallbladder, and pancreas. The GI tract resembles a long tube that begins from the mouth and ends in the anus. When we eat food, it goes through this tube where it is broken down, and all the nutrients in the food are absorbed into the bloodstream. Finally, any indigestible remains are expelled from the body as feces.

The digestion of food starts in the mouth. Your mouth will begin to produce saliva in anticipation of the food by smelling your favourite meal. Saliva contains an enzyme called *amylase*, which breaks down carbohydrates into glucose. As the food enters the mouth and mixes with the saliva, the carbs will be broken down before getting to the stomach. Saliva also moistens the chewed food for easy swallowing.

Once the food is swallowed, it'll move into the throat or pharynx (another structure in the GI tract) before entering the esophagus (a structure in the GI tract). The esophagus is a muscular tube that connects the throat to the stomach. Muscles in the esophagus contract to create a wave called peristalsis that moves the food down to the stomach.

Upon entering the stomach (another structure in the GI tract), a muscular ring at the end of the esophagus called the sphincter immediately shuts to prevent the food or fluid from flowing back into the esophagus. In the stomach, the food is churned and mixed with digestive juices with acid and enzymes, which help further to break down the food into much smaller pieces. This mixing processes the food into a thick liquid called chyme. The chyme won't leave the stomach until it has reached the right consistency to pass into the small intestine. The chyme is squirted down into the small intestine from the stomach, where digestion continues, and nutrients are absorbed from the food into the bloodstream.

The small intestine is a GI structure made up of three parts: duodenum, jejunum, ileum. Duodenum is the first part of the small intestine connected to the stomach. The jejunum is the coiled midsection of the small intestine, while the ileum is the last part of the small intestine that leads into the large intestine. It's in these structures that vitamins, minerals, glucose, fatty acids, amino acids, and water are absorbed from the chyme to be used by all your other body systems.

Accessory structures such as the liver,

pancreas, and gallbladder are essential to digestion. The liver makes a substance called bile that helps the body absorb fat. Bile is stored in the gallbladder until it is needed. The pancreas produces all the enzymes the small intestine uses to digest carbs, protein, and fat. Any undigested material in the small intestine is moved to the large intestine.

The large intestine is also a GI structure that helps the body absorb water from the undigested remains, which changes the waste from liquid to solid. The solid waste (feces) then moves via peristalsis from the large intestine to the rectum, where they're stored. The stool is then expelled from the rectum through the anus (the final structure in the GI tract) during a bowel movement.

Our digestive system needs to be healthy for these processes to occur efficiently. You can know if your digestive system is healthy by how regular and frequent your bowel movements are. If it's working well, you can expect to have at least two to three bowel movements a day. So for your digestive system to work efficiently, eat foods rich in fibre. Fibre helps absorb water, solidifying and bulking your stool, making it easier to pass out of the body. Fibre-rich foods include fruits, whole grains, and vegetables. In addition, other foods like yogurts, tempeh, kefir, kombucha, fennel, and chia seeds are excellent at improving digestion.

- **Circulatory/cardiovascular system**

The circulatory system, also known as the cardiovascular system, comprises the heart, the blood, and the blood vessels. Blood vessels include arteries, veins, and capillaries. The circulatory system carries blood to all parts of your body. Blood helps to transport nutrients and oxygen throughout the body while picking up waste from your cells and organs to be expelled from the body. The wastes are the carbon dioxide gas from respiration, chemical by-products from your cells and organs, and the unwanted substances from the things you eat and drink.

The heart lies at the focal point of the circulatory system. It pumps the blood, but the transport of blood away from and toward the heart occurs through the blood vessels. As a result, your arteries carry blood rich in oxygen and nutrients from the heart to the rest of your body. By contrast, your veins carry oxygen and nutrient-poor blood from your cells and organs back to the heart. The capillaries, however, are very tiny blood vessels that connect the arteries to the veins. At the capillaries, carbon dioxide is exchanged for oxygen and nutrients.

The heart is one of the most complex organs in your body. It consists of four chambers: the left and right atriums located at the top of the heart and the left and right ventricles from the bottom chambers. The two atria receive the blood entering the heart, while the two ventricles carry blood out of the heart. In addition, one-way valves separate the top and bottom chambers to ensure blood flows in the right direction.

When oxygen in the blood depletes, for example, veins carry it to the heart's right atrium during physical activity. Then it's pumped by the right ventricle into the lungs, where it receives oxygen. From the lungs, the oxygenated blood flows back toward the heart. It enters the heart from the left atrium then flows to the left ventricle before being pumped and carried throughout the body through the arteries. This circulation process repeats itself to keep your organs, tissues, and muscles healthy.

A healthy heart pumps blood at the right amount needed for your body to function. If the right amount of blood is jeopardized due to diseases or injury to your heart, your cells and organs will not receive enough blood to work normally. So to maintain proper blood volume, stay hydrated and ensure you're getting enough potassium from your diet. Likewise, eat foods rich in folate, iron, copper, and vitamin B12 to make more hemoglobin, which helps form more red blood cells.

It's normal to lose some blood when you have a cut or injury. But excessive amounts can be dangerous. For instance, when we sustain an injury, our body activates an internal mechanism that causes our blood to clot. Blood clotting is a natural response to preventing excessive bleeding. In this process, our blood will change from a liquid to a gel-like state to reduce blood loss. In addition, blood clotting helps us maintain a healthy blood volume. So to prevent excessive bleeding, a diet that's rich in vitamins K and E can help you conserve your blood.

Other foods that can increase blood flow include cayenne pepper, onions, garlic, cinnamon, ginger, turmeric, and fatty fish.

- **Nervous system**

The nervous system comprises the brain, spinal cord, and nerve. It controls many processes in our body, like our thoughts, emotions, and feelings. Even the things our body does, such as digestion, breathing, heart rate, sexual development, blinking, and movements, are regulated by our nervous system. As a result, it affects every aspect of our health.

The nervous system is divided into the central nervous system (CNS) and the peripheral nervous system (PNS). The CNS is made up of the brain and spinal cord. Information in the form of electrical signals is sent to our brain, where they're analyzed and interpreted, preparing our body for an adequate response. Our nerves help send information to and from different parts of our body. The brain and the spinal cord have nerves branching off to other parts of our body. These nerves make up our PNS. The PNS helps to carry information to other parts of our body. Once the information in our brain is interpreted, it communicates with the spinal cord through neural pathways before the information is sent to the rest of our body through the PNS. The nerves that carry information from the brain to other body parts are called efferent neurons. Our bodies respond by causing us to either "fight or flight" or "rest and digest."

These two divisions of the nervous system communicate with themselves to help us interpret what's going on around us and respond appropriately. For example, when faced with an external threat, the information is automatically sent to our brain, where it is interpreted as either life-threatening or not. The nerves that carry information from other body parts to our CNS are afferent neurons. If our brain interprets it as life-threatening, we immediately enter a fight or flight mode. But when the threat is no more, our body goes into a rest and digest state to help us relax.

Our peripheral nervous system comprises two subsystems: somatic and autonomic nervous systems. The somatic nervous system controls our voluntary actions using our skeletal muscles. These are things we do consciously while being fully aware such as moving our legs and walking. Our nervous system controls involuntary heart rate, digestion, respiration, etc. But they occur through the autonomic nervous system.

The autonomic nervous system is subdivided into the sympathetic nervous system (responsible for our fight or flight response) and the parasympathetic nervous system (responsible for our rest and digest response). If the sympathetic nervous system is activated, our body will prevent the parasympathetic nervous system from becoming activated and vice versa.

All the bodily processes our nervous system regulates can weigh it down if it isn't properly cared for. The good news is that you can do simple things to rejuvenate and maintain the nerves working together. One of such ways is to feed yourself nutritious foods. Seriously, our brain and our nervous system love a balanced diet. Foods rich in vitamins B1 and B12 are essential in maintaining our nervous system. These nutrients can be found in eggs, fish, chicken, legumes, meat, almonds, and spinach.

Moreover, since glucose is the primary

energy source for our brains, a diet containing complex carbohydrates like whole grains and starchy vegetables can provide our brains with a steadier energy source. Our brain and nervous system also love fat, but in healthy amounts. Fats from avocado, nuts, seeds, and fatty fish can protect us against neurological diseases and are required for proper brain function.

Likewise, our nervous system needs nutrients like magnesium, calcium, potassium, and sodium to enable our nerves to communicate with each other effectively.

- **Lymphatic system**

The lymphatic system is part of our immune system. It consists of lymphatic vessels, lymph, and collecting ducts. One of the primary functions of our lymphatic system is to drain excess fluids called lymph from tissues in our body and return them to the blood. How does this extra fluid form? The liquid part of our blood, known as the plasma, helps carry nutrients, hormones, and proteins to the rest of our body. So when our heart pumps blood, it delivers nutrients to our cells and organs and receives their waste in the process. During this exchange, some plasma seeps through the capillaries into our body tissues, where they're stored as lymph.

Besides nutrients and other substances that nourish our body, lymph may contain foreign particles like bacteria, viruses, damaged cells, or cancerous cells that may have been trapped by the fluids between our cells. The lymphatic vessels drain the lymph and return it to our bloodstream through the collecting ducts. We have lots of lymph vessels throughout our bodies. They're bigger than capillaries but smaller than veins. If the lymph isn't drained, the excess fluid can build up and cause our body tissues to swell, leading to edema.

There are two major collecting ducts in our body: the left and right lymphatic ducts. The left lymphatic duct, also known as the thoracic duct, starts close to the lower part of our spine and runs up through the chest. It gathers lymph from our lower chest area, pelvis, and abdomen and discharges it into our blood through a large vein near the left side of our neck. The right lymphatic duct gathers lymph from the right side of our neck, arm, and chest and discharges it into our blood through a large vein near the right side of our neck. By returning the lymph to our bloodstream, we're able to maintain our blood pressure and volume in a healthy range.

Our lymphatic system also helps to protect us against disease-causing organisms. There are structures in the lymphatic system known as lymph nodes that help to filter and cleanse the lymph. Lymph nodes are glands located all over the body. They filter damaged cells and cancer cells from the blood that may be present in the lymph. Lymph nodes also produce and store white blood cells (lymphocytes) and other immune cells used to destroy bacteria and other substances in the lymph. We have a collection of lymph nodes in our neck, groin, and armpit areas. The lymph nodes are where many immune reactions are initiated. So when you're ill, doctors typically check for swollen lymph nodes. Swelling signals an infection.

Your lymphatic system plays a massive role in your health and overall well-being. But, since it's tied to your immune and circulatory systems, you can easily ignore or forget about it. Only remember it when you become sick and have problems with your lymph nodes. However, you can start today to treat your lymphatic system better by eating foods like leafy greens, nuts and seeds, citrus fruits, turmeric, ginger, garlic, and drinking lots of water to boost the lymphatic system. A healthy lymphatic system will be more efficient at removing sources of pain, aches, and excess fat from the body.

- **Respiratory system**

Our respiratory system is what allows us to breathe in and out. It requires oxygen to function, enabling us to take in oxygen and remove carbon dioxide gas from our bodies while breathing out. This movement of carbon dioxide and oxygen is called respiration. Without the respiratory system, we also won't be able to talk and smell nor protect our airways from irritants and other harmful substances.

Our respiratory system is made up of structures such as the mouth, pharynx (or throat), voice box (or larynx), nose, lungs, and windpipe (or trachea), which work together to enable us to breathe.

Air enters our respiratory system through our mouth or nose and passes down the throat through the voice box. If air enters through the nose, it is warmed. The tiny hairs in our nose, called *cilia,* filter the air before it passes down to the voice box. Air coming into the body, through the mouth and nose, meet at the pharynx before it's delivered to the windpipe. The pharynx has two openings: one for the passage of food and the other for the passage of air. The pathway for food leads to the stomach, while that for air leads to the lungs. Typically, one pathway closes when the other is active. For example, if you're about to swallow food or liquid, the air passage is covered by a small tissue to prevent the food and liquid from entering the lungs. From the pharynx, the air moves through the voice box to the windpipe. In the windpipe, cilia are lined all around the walls to sweep fluids and foreign particles out of the air that'd enter the lungs. Once air enters the lungs, they inflate, and when the air leaves the lungs, they deflate.

Your ribs and diaphragm also help you breathe in and out. When you breathe in, your diaphragm moves downwards toward your abdomen, and the muscles in your ribs pull your ribs upwards and outwards. This makes your chest walls increase and become more extensive, pulling the air into your lungs. But when you exhale, your diaphragm moves upwards, and your rib muscles pull the ribs downward and inwards. This subsequently causes the walls of your chest to decrease and become smaller, pushing the air out of your respiratory system through your mouth or nose. With each inhalation, oxygen and carbon dioxide are exchanged in tiny air sacs in the lungs called alveoli. Then the oxygen is picked up by the blood and pumped through our arteries to other parts of our body.

Any abnormality in our airways affects our overall health. Fortunately, we can improve the functioning of every organ and structure that makes up the respiratory system by eating healthy foods. Foods rich in flavonoids, beta carotene, omega-3 fatty acids, and vitamins C and E can help to keep our lungs healthy. These nutrients can be found in foods like beet and beet greens, dark leafy greens, apples, turmeric, blueberries, tomatoes and their products, fatty fish, olive oil, Brazil nuts, red cabbage, and pumpkins.

- **Urinary system**

OUR URINARY SYSTEM helps us remove excess salt, extra water, and toxins from our blood through our urine. Other vital functions of our urinary system are to balance our body's pH, regulate our blood pressure, and control the number of electrolytes (such as chlorine, calcium, potassium, magnesium, and sodium) in our blood. It's made up of one urethra, one bladder, two ureters, and two kidneys.

Our kidneys play two essential roles in our body: filter waste from the blood and produce urine. You might be wondering where the waste in the blood comes from. During the process of digestion, lots of waste products are generated. Your body will separate the nutrients you need from the toxins by filtering the blood. If the kidneys do not remove these harmful substances from our blood, they can build up and make us sick. Generally, we should aim to keep the two kidneys in good health, but if one of them becomes damaged or fails, we can still survive on just one kidney. Doctors can use your urine sample to tell how healthy your kidneys are and how much water you have in your body. For example, if white blood cells are found in your urine, it's a sign of an infection. Likewise, the colour of your urine says a lot about how hydrated you are. If you drink a lot of water, your urine will be pale yellow. Conversely, a dehydrated body produces urine that's dark yellow.

Once your kidneys produce urine, it is moved through the ureters to your bladder, where it is stored. Waste products equally move to your bladder once your blood has been filtered. Your bladder can hold urine until you're ready to urinate. It's shaped like a balloon and made of muscle. Your bladder expands as more waste and urine are produced and stored. Once your bladder is full, nerves in your bladder will signal to your brain that you need to urinate. When you're ready to urinate, your bladder will contract, and the muscle that controls exit from the bladder will relax to allow the contents of your bladder to come out. Waste products and urine then flow out of the bladder through the urethra to the outside environment. The urethra for women is in front of the vaginal opening, while that of men stops at the tip of the penis.

We need every structure and organ in our respiratory system to remain healthy and disease-free. With a nutritious diet, our kidneys will properly control our blood sugar and blood pressure, which will lower our risk for any kidney disease. If the bulk of your diet consists of salty and sugar foods, high blood sugar levels and high blood pressure can damage the blood vessels in our kidneys and make it less efficient at filtering our blood. So a diet rich in whole, unprocessed foods and lean meat will prevent elevated blood pressure and sugar levels.

Our kidneys balance the pH of our blood using the electrolytes (magnesium, sodium, potassium, and water) found in our blood to adjust the pH back to a healthy range. So eating foods rich in these nutrients can keep our body's acid-base levels balanced. Foods such as beet and beet greens, carrots, lentils, cabbage, tomatoes, blueberries, and spinach are excellent sources of these nutrients.

A NUTRIENT-RICH BODY IS A HEALTHY BODY

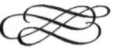

A nourished body does more than just keep you energized. It fights diseases, kills cancer cells, heals wounds, and combats aging. The body can restore itself to health under the right conditions quickly. Unfortunately, we don't typically engage our body's built-in health mechanisms when we become sick. Instead, we assume it has failed us and turn to medications. Besides eating a healthy diet, some of us aren't aware of other ways to enhance our body's natural health capacity.

The human body has a variety of ways of helping itself. When our cells rupture; become damaged due to injury from normal wear-

and-tear, all the components and organelles within the cell spill out. A damaged cell must repair itself. To do so, the cell will first stop things from spilling out of it and then regenerate itself by rebuilding and replacing those missing or damaged components.

A typical example is when you have a cut on your skin. After you cut the skin, tiny cells circulate in your blood called platelets to help your body form clots to stop the bleeding. Then a scab forms over that area before attracting white blood cells to the site of the injury. White blood cells protect the wounded area from germs. Immediately the immune cells are recruited, all the dead cells are removed, and the injured cells are repaired. This is how our bodies constantly remove damaged cells to produce new healthier ones.

The body also uses stem cells to help regenerate itself. Stem cells can develop into any cell in the body. They're used to replace cells and tissues that have been damaged or lost due to illnesses. For example, stem cells can be found in the body of an embryo that is three to five days old. As the embryo is being formed in the womb, the stem cells begin to grow and divide to form different cells necessary to develop properly.

Even as adults, stem cells are in our bone marrow. However, these stem cells divide only to form a specific cell type. For instance, epithelial stem cells can only regenerate cells in the skin; neural stem cells can only regenerate nerve cells in the brain and spinal cord; and mesenchymal stem cells can regenerate bone cells, muscle cells, fat cells, and cartilage cells. So if your physician, for example, wants to treat your damaged muscle cells, they can transplant mesenchymal stem cells into your muscle to produce new muscle cells.

Likewise, our immune system attacks intruders such as bacteria, fungi, and viruses to keep us healthy and fight any ongoing illness. For example, white blood cells called leukocytes patrol our blood and tissue, searching for foreign substances. When our white blood cells encounter a target, they send signals to other immune cells, which activates the immune response. Immune cells like phagocytes (a type of white blood cell) then engulf and destroy the invader. If the intruder is a virus, white blood cells called natural killer cells eliminate cells that the virus has infected.

Our bodies can sometimes trigger an inflammatory response when it's reacting to an injury or infection, activating our immune system. An example of an inflammatory response is a fever. Your body can fight pathogens by causing you to have a fever. Fever increases our body's temperature too high enough levels to stimulate leukocytes to kill the pathogens. Most bacteria and viruses thrive when our bodies are at a normal temperature. But a fever makes it difficult for pathogens to survive.

Tools to Improve Your Body's Ability Towards Better Health

The following factors play an essential role in allowing the body to help itself from the inside out and stay in a harmonious state.

- **Nutrition:** We all need food to survive. Food is one of the necessities of life that nobody can live without. Without food, people will die. Our cells and organs depend on what we eat to thrive. It supplies us the energy and nutrients to go about our daily lives. Food plays a massive role in our overall well-being. If you deprive your body of the vitamins, minerals, and other nutrients needed to flourish, you can predispose yourself to malnutrition and other illnesses. This is essential because what we eat is key to our well-being.

Food is a huge component of holistic nutrition. It gives our bodies the materials and information to function effectively. What we eat can be medicinal and help maintain health and prevent illnesses. The nutrients in what we eat, power all the essential bodily functions. They are required to grow, develop, and maintain these internal processes. Nutrients are so essential that without them, our health will decline. It's just as important to consume them in the right amounts. Our bodies require different amounts of different nutrients. And when we don't meet our nutritional needs, our biological processes can slow down or cease. In other words, nutrients guide our bodies on how to function.

Diets focusing on a single nutrient can cause you to consume high amounts of one nutrient, which increases your risk for health problems. These foods are typically nutrient-poor but high in calories and sodium, saturated fat, and added sugars, e.g., sweets, sweetened beverages, and other processed foods. We need to balance nutrients in our diets to reap health benefits.

Some nutrients influence how other nutrients are absorbed in the body. For example, iron helps our bodies absorb vitamin C. There are two forms of iron: heme and nonheme iron. Heme iron is found in animal protein sources and is easily absorbed by the body. But nonheme iron, found in plant protein sources, is difficult for our bodies to absorb without vitamin C in the diet. Legumes, grains, nuts, and seeds all contain a compound known as phytate or phytic acid that can prevent the absorption of iron, zinc, and calcium.

. . .

So what can you do? You can change your cooking technique to remove some acid from your food. Soaking your grains, legumes, and seeds before cooking them will decrease the amount of phytic acid in your diet. Then consume your plant protein sources together with vitamin-c rich foods to increase iron absorption. By reducing the amount of phytic acid, you're also helping your body absorb calcium and zinc.

Moreover, certain foods need fat to be absorbed. Foods rich in carotenoids and fat-soluble vitamins such as vitamins A, D, E, and K, need to be consumed with fat for absorption. Carotenoids are compounds produced by plants that give them their respective colours. You can find them in red, yellow, orange, and dark-green vegetables. If you consume these vegetables without any source of fat—for example, eating salad with a fat-free dressing—you may be missing out on vital nutrients. Pairing foods rich in carotenoids and fat-soluble vitamins with healthy fats like avocados, nuts, or olive oil will equally increase the nutritional content of the food.

Likewise, foods like seeds, vegetables, nuts,

fruits, and cocoa contain a compound called oxalate (or oxalic acids) that prevents the absorption of calcium and iron when combined with fibre. This is because oxalate binds to calcium or iron in our diet to form compounds like calcium oxalate and iron oxalate. By doing so, our gut won't absorb calcium and iron from our diets. For example, spinach is a rich source of calcium and oxalate, which prevents a lot of the calcium from being absorbed. However, you can increase calcium absorption by eating dairy products such as milk together with oxalate-containing foods. The calcium absorption from dairy products is not affected when combined with oxalate-containing foods.

Multiple studies have traced chronic illnesses to our dietary choices. Undernutrition is just as bad as overnutrition. For example, insufficient intake of vitamin A increases your risk for vision problems both in adults and children. But in children, it's more harmful because it can cause childhood blindness. Other nutrients like iron can cause anemia when our bodies aren't getting it in sufficient amounts.

- **Sleep:** To be asleep means to be in a state where your body is at rest and your nervous system is inactive, causing you to be temporarily unconscious. However, our brains are still active during sleep doing important things. There are different stages of sleep: In the first stage, we're slightly asleep, but our brains are still processing information. So a little noise around you can wake you up. The second stage of sleep is somewhat deeper than the first stage, and noises around you may not easily wake you up. Once you enter the third stage, you're deeply asleep, and it is more difficult to wake up. Also, if this stage of sleep is interrupted, it may be harder to go back to sleep. The fourth stage of sleep is known as REM sleep. This is when we dream.

Sleep is essential for your well-being. Numerous studies have noted that the amount of sleep you get can affect the functioning of your brain, your body, and your health. So how much sleep do we need? The length of sleep differs from person to person, but on average, it's recommended that adults get seven to nine hours of sleep, while teenagers, babies, and young children need more than nine hours of sleep for growth and development.

Sufficient sleep and the lack thereof can impact your body in so many ways:

- **It affects your ability to learn and remember:** Anytime you learn new information, new neural pathways are created in your brain. When the information is needed, your brain can tap into our long-term memory to retrieve the information. Each of these steps is necessary for proper brain processing. Sleep processes the new information and seals our memory. It strengthens the neural networks in the brain that form our memories. So when you're well-rested, you're more able to remember all you learned while awake. That means staying awake all night to learn new information wouldn't help you better remember it the same way you would have if you were well-rested.

Sleep plays a significant role in our ability to focus, pay attention, and learn new information. Adequate sleep helps to keep our attention and focus sharp. However, it isn't easy to be vigilant and attentive when sleep-deprived, making learning new information challenging. In addition, without sufficient sleep, our nerves may no longer properly coordinate information, and we may find it challenging to recall information.

- **It affects your mood**: You probably have firsthand experience of what sleep deprivation can do to your mood. Sleep helps to regulate our emotions. When you don't get sufficient sleep, you may be more short-tempered, irritable, and easily susceptible to stress. But once you sleep well, your mood brightens up, and you often return to normal. Mood imbalance due to low-quality sleep has consequences for learning.

Alterations in mood affect our ability to acquire new information and remember it.

Not only does the quantity of sleep affect your mood, but your mood can equally affect your sleep. Mood disorders like anxiety increase arousal and agitation, making it difficult to sleep. Conversely, sleep deprivation boosts a part of our brain that's often affected by mood disorders. So chronic insomnia increases your risk for developing mood problems like depression, anxiety, and other psychiatric problems.

- **It influences your health:** Many changes go on in your body when you sleep. Your heart rate decreases, body temperature drops, and your kidneys slow down the rate of urine production. That's why you don't feel the urge to urinate as frequently as you would when you're awake. Sleep is also the time when your body produces more growth hormones and other hormones that control your appetite. Growth hormone helps to rejuvenate our skin, makes our hair grow longer, and helps kids grow taller.

Sleep boosts your immune system and your body's ability to fight diseases. When we're asleep, our bodies produce more anti-inflammatory proteins known as cytokines to fight inflammation and free radicals in the body. Sleep is the time when our bodies release hormones and proteins to repair damaged tissues and blood vessels. But if you're sleep-deprived, your body will heal more slowly.

Insufficient sleep has been linked to numerous health problems like premature death, obesity, hypertension, cardiovascular disease, and diabetes. For instance, eating foods high in calories with little to no exercise is a risk factor for obesity. However, insufficient sleep increases your appetite. Your appetite is controlled by two hormones- ghrelin and leptin. Ghrelin increases the feelings of hunger while leptin suppresses it. Adequate sleep balances the levels of these two hormones in your body throughout the day. However, being behind on sleep creates an imbalance in these hormones, causing your body to produce more ghrelin. As such, you may consume more calories than you usually would have on a well-rested day.

- **Exercise:** Nutrition is more than just the nutrients we give our bodies. It includes physical activity and how it helps us maintain our health and prevent diseases. Exercise reduces our risk for type-2 diabetes, obesity, and cardiovascular diseases. It provides both immediate and long-term health benefits. There are two forms of exercise: endurance and resistance exercise.

Endurance exercise (a.k.a. aerobic exercises) like walking, swimming, running, cycling, and so on that can help you shed pounds. You can perform it at different intensities. During the exercise, your heart rate and breathing increase. This exercise can help you burn belly fat, a risk factor for type-2 diabetes and heart disease.

Resistance exercises, however, enable you to build your muscles. We commonly know this form of exercise as strength training or weight training. It requires you to make your muscles work against a weight or force to build strength and increase muscle mass. You can perform resistance exercises using weight machines, your body weight, resistance bands, and free weights. The more muscle mass you have, the higher your metabolism and the more fat you'll burn.

To enjoy all the health benefits of exercise, researchers and health professionals recommend at least 30 minutes of moderately intense exercise daily.

Besides your weight, regular exercise is good for your mind. If you suffer from depression, performing physical activity may help you think more positive thoughts and take your mind off your worries. Depression can manifest itself physically in the form of loss of appetite, body pains, fatigue, reduced energy, and difficulty sleeping, all of which can make you loose motivation to exercise. But getting up and moving helps combat depression. Your body releases feel-good hormones when you perform high-intensity exercises. However, you can benefit more by performing moderate-intensity exercises.

Moderate-intensity activities stimulate our brains to release proteins called neurotrophic or growth factors, which causes nerve cells in our brains to grow and form new connections. In the region of our brain that controls our mood, nerve cell growth improves the functioning of our brains, which helps to relieve depression.

Exercising around other people increases your chances of interacting and creating social networks, which is healthy for your mind. It's one thing to begin to exercise, but it's another thing to maintain interest and stay motivated. Exercising around others is more fun, and you're less likely to get bored. It serves as a shared interest, making it easier to bond with others. Over time, it'll be easier to converse about other things and get to know people. You may share jokes, laugh, and encourage each other during and after your exercise, which is healthy for you. Laughter is good for the mind and body. It activates multiple regions of your brain, strengthening neural connections. A great way to broaden your friendship group is by joining an exercise class.

What's more, regular exercise is a good

stress management technique. Too much stress can cause our muscles and joints to tense up, causing body pains. While exercising, your body releases more of its natural painkillers and mood elevators. This helps to relax and calm our nerves. In addition, exercises like meditation, breathing exercises, and yoga activate our parasympathetic nervous system and inhibit the sympathetic nervous system—your heart rate and blood pressure decrease from bringing your body to a calm state. As you enter a state of deep relaxation, your body enhances the activities of your immune cells, making it easier to fight illnesses and diseases.

Yoga exercises like *asanas* can strengthen your heart muscles to pump more blood throughout your body and improve your body's ability to use oxygen. Both of these changes positively impact your overall health. In addition, it protects your heart against cardiovascular problems.

Other body systems like the respiratory system improve during exercise. Your lungs will function properly, and you'll find relief from stress. Whatever your source of stress is, exercising helps distract the mind and refocuses it on the task at hand. It's relaxing and calming to your body.

- **Stress:** Stress is a major component of your body being in an imbalance. It affects your body's ability to help itself if it isn't properly managed. Whether emotional, physical, or occupational stress, all forms of stress can reduce your body's resiliency and delay the feel good process. How our bodies respond to stress depends on our genes, presence or absence of a support system (family and/or friends), your personality, and your coping mechanisms. Multiple studies have noted that people with stronger social support systems tend to manage stress better and are more resilient than those without.

Using the stress bucket analogy, you can measure how much stress your body can tolerate. This imaginary bucket consists of both your short and long-term stressors. As you add more stressors to the bucket, it fills up to a level where it begins to overflow. At this point, you've experienced too much stress than your body can tolerate. Our bodies use physical, emotional, or behavioural signs to tell us that we're experiencing too much stress. By listening to your body closely, you can quickly notice any signs and then begin to reduce or release your stress. Unfortunately, the size of our stress buckets varies from person to person, and we cannot change it. However, you can adopt coping strategies to prevent your bucket from overflowing.

A more sustainable way to manage stress is by committing to daily copying techniques to help reduce stress. Reducing your stress levels is one of the most critical factors in allowing your body to stay in its harmonious state. Here is a list of a few things you can do:

- **Reduce your obligations and commitments**: Life is full of endless opportunities, but our bodies can only endure so much. Focusing on only the most important commitments will significantly reduce your stressors. Sometimes you must set boundaries and draw the line on how far you're willing to devote yourself to something. This will help you fully commit and be more productive with a few obligations. You can equally share your responsibilities to reduce the load. Essentially, don't bite off more than you can chew. You can avoid overcommitting by examining your schedule to know how much time you can realistically devote to a task. It is equally important to learn to say "yes" or "no" when necessary.

- **Exercise:** Regularly performing mind-focusing exercises like praying, meditation, and guided imagery can teach you how to focus your mind. These exercises train your brain to only concentrate on whatever you're doing at that time. Prayer also has the same effect on your brain. People have historically been using prayer to reduce their anxiety levels, manage pain, and improve overall health—likewise, guided imagery. Guided imagery is a relaxation tool that encourages you to focus on positive thoughts only. It has been proven to reduce mood disorders, pain and improve sleep.

Other relation techniques like yoga and talk therapy are equally good at lowering stress. Yoga is a form of exercise. It combines different alternative health methods such as postural exercises, breathing exercises, meditation, and guided imagery. However, deep breathing and stretching exercises are best for lowering stress. During deep breathing, your body enters a state of deep rest that can alter how your body responds to stress. Your brain receives more oxygen in this state, and all the physiological reactions triggered by the sympathetic nervous system calm down.

- **Herbal remedies:** Some herbs can strengthen a stressed-out body. Herbs like *Rhodiola Rosea, Panax ginseng,* and *Eleutherococcus senticosus* can help reduce your stress. These herbs support the functioning of your adrenal glands. Adrenal glands produce hormones that regulate how your body responds to stress. So these herbs help to balance the number of stress hormones in your blood, thereby increasing your body's resilience to stress to help you recover. Other herbs like lemon balm, passionflower, Bacopa, valerian, chamomile, and hops stimulate our brain to release high amounts of hormones to help us relax.

You can consume these herbs as tea or supplements. And you can add some to your baths or enjoy their benefits through essential oils.

THE FIVE ASPECTS OF HOLISTIC HEALTH

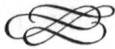

*H*olistic health encompasses every aspect of a person's life, such as physical health, emotional health, social health, mental health and spiritual health. Each dimension of wellness works together to influence your overall well-being. This approach to wellness depends on greater factors than simply not showing obvious symptoms of illness. So begin to evaluate your holistic health and well-being on a much broader spectrum.

There's no one-sit-fits-all approach to holistic health. Every individual's path to wellness is unique, and it's affected by external and internal factors such as your diet, personality, environment, and genes. That's why you need to personalize your care.

Dimensions of Wellness

Let's learn more about holistic health and its importance in our overall well-being.

1. Physical health

Our physical body is what most people think about when they think of being healthy. It can show visible signs of illness, making it easier to monitor and treat. The health of our physical body is a function of how well we've been taking care of it. If you can't do little things like walking, standing for a few minutes, and lifting, you may not be taking proper care of your body. Our physical body is an essential part of who we are.

The state of our bodies has a profound impact on our minds and emotions. Our physical and emotional health are much more connected than many people recognize. Our feelings are intensified by how we feel about ourselves physically. For instance, a deformity in the face can make you sad and rouse negative thoughts in your mind. Likewise, mood disorders like depression and anxiety can be heightened or directly caused by physical ailments. This means that merely taking care of your physical appearance can help improve your emotional health. And this, in turn, can boost your self-esteem and confidence level, which may help prevent negative emotions and mood disorders.

Self-esteem is your negative or positive evaluation of how you see yourself, what you think you're good at, who you are, and what your strengths and weaknesses may be. Low self-esteem is accompanied by negative emotions such as depression and anxiety. These negative emotions lead to bad behaviours like smoking and alcohol abuse. The more a person indulges in these unhealthy behaviours, the more their physical body deteriorates. Smoking, for instance, damages our skin and accelerates ageing.

On the other hand, a high level of self-esteem is followed by positive emotions such as relaxation, gratitude, delight, optimism, and joy. So there's a direct connection between our health and our attitude. When you're healthy, it is easier to be optimistic. So starting a healthy lifestyle might be easier for you.

Our physical bodies can even influence our ability to reason and make sound decisions. We all know that regular physical activity can improve how we look. But did you know it's equally good for your mental health? Yes, getting busy working your muscles benefits your brain! Regular exercise helps to improve the functioning of our brain and slow down age-related loss in our ability to think, reason, and create memories. It does this by triggering the release of hormones that support the growth of new brain cells and stimulating new neural connections in our brain. Exercise equally helps your heart pump more blood to your brain, which is necessary for your brain functioning.

Likewise, taking care of our physical bodies impacts our energy levels throughout the day. Eating healthy foods to help you manage your weight directly boosts your energy levels. They provide your body with the nutrients it needs to function well. Whole foods, healthy fats, and lean meat can increase your satiety and keep you energized for more extended periods. In addition, movements like stretching and walking are energy-boosting activities that help reduce stress and calm you down.

You can improve the functioning of your physical body (and your mental and emotional health) by eating nutritious foods, getting sufficient sleep, regularly exercising, and eliminating unhealthy lifestyles like smoking.

2. Emotional health

Our emotional well-being is just as crucial as our physical health. They're closely interconnected, and both influence one another—every human experience various emotions that influence our lives, interactions with others, and overall health. Six basic emotions are universal: disgust, surprise, happiness, anger, sadness, and fear.

- **Disgust:** We express disgust by turning away from the source of revulsion, vomiting, and wrinkling our nose. This emotion can originate from perceiving a foul

smell or an unpleasant taste or sight. What people find disgusting can also vary from culture to culture (such as certain types of food). For instance, eating fish can be disgusting to a person who doesn't eat seafood. We develop this emotion from a young age. Between the ages of four to eight, children begin to express disgust toward things they find repulsive. Disgust serves a fundamental purpose in our lives. It keeps us away from things that are dangerous or potentially damaging.
- **Happiness:** Of all the six basic emotions, happiness is the emotion that we strive for the most. Happiness is your ability to be joyful, satisfied, and content at any time.

When someone is happy, you can tell from their facial expressions, body language, and the tone of their voice. A happy person has a smile on their face and relaxed body language. The things that contribute to happiness vary from person to person. Happiness is good for our mental and physical health. It lowers our risk for type-2 diabetes, cardiovascular diseases, mood disorders, and mental health problems.

- **Surprise**: When you react to something unexpected, you're exhibiting this emotion. Surprise can be a negative or positive reaction. A positive surprise will be someone giving you an item you've always wanted. You may react by yelling, gasping, or screaming when you're surprised. You may show facial expressions like opening your mouth, raising your brows, and widening your eyes. Some people jump back when they're surprised. Surprise, whether positive or negative, triggers a fight or flight response. We may experience an adrenaline rush that prepares us to fight or flee when startled.
- **Anger**: This is one of those strong emotions that, if not properly

managed, can be harmful to your health. We often show anger through the tone of our voice, aggressive behaviours, facial expressions, body language, or physiological responses like turning red or sweating. Despite the negative connotation of this emotion, there are times when being angry can benefit you. It can help you clarify your help in a relationship and equally motivate you to solve your problems. It's ok to express your anger, but it can become a problem when expressed in unhealthy, harmful, and dangerous ways. If you can't control your anger, you can quickly become violent, aggressive, or abusive, detrimental to your physical and mental health. People who are quick to anger may have difficulties making rational decisions.

- **Sadness**: Everyone experiences sadness from time to time. Sadness is an emotional state where we feel disappointed, hopeless, and in a low mood. And it can last for either a short or long-time. Prolonged and severe sadness negatively impacts your mental health and leads to depression. It can cause you to engage in unhealthy coping behaviours like ruminating on negative thoughts, isolating yourself from others, and self-medicating. These behaviours can prolong and exacerbate sadness.

EVERYONE HAS a unique way of coping with sadness, and there are telltale signs to know someone is sad. For example, withdrawal from others, unusual quietness, crying, lethargy, or low mood is typically expressed when we're sad.

Other types of emotions include embarrassment, excitement, pride, and shame. Being healthy emotionally plays an essential role in fostering self-awareness and resilience. Resilience is your ability to bounce back from adversities. While adversities are undoubtedly sad, they don't have to define who you are. Becoming resilient helps you take control and modify certain aspects of your life. That's not to say you'll never have any negative emotions. But having good emotional health gives you the ability to manage difficulties every day.

Working on your emotional health is important. It helps you to build resilience to stress. Being resilient during stressful situations is not about avoiding or resisting stress but developing effective coping strategies. No matter how robust our resilience is, we'll always encounter stress. So it's crucial to develop resilience. It can take time to build resilience to stress. A lot of soul searching, daily practice, and evaluating your values and the reasons for doing what you do go into developing stress resilience. Resilience is beneficial for our mental health. It can help protect you from various mental health conditions like anxiety and depression. It can equally reduce your risk of developing mental health problems from past traumatic events.

3. Social health

Humans are social creatures. Our brains have evolved to require social interactions to function well. Our social health is measured by the quality of relationships with others around us. Since the day we were born, we have required connections to assist us with figuring out how to explore our environment. Social links with family, friends and the community are necessary for our overall well-being. They serve as support systems that can carry us through difficult situations. Don't underestimate the power of surrounding yourself with people who care about you. You need to be able to turn to someone for support when necessary.

Various research has shown that forming deep connections helps us live happy lives.

THE COOL THING about regularly interacting with others is that it helps strengthen your social skills, which are required to build emotionally supportive networks to stay mentally and physically healthy. When you're healthy socially, you'll be able to form meaningful relationships. Don't limit yourself to a small demographic as you develop your social skills. Expand your horizon to people from diverse settings. It's important to have the ability to relate to others of different backgrounds and life experiences.

Being part of a community can help improve your well-being outside your friends and family. This is why belonging to a religious group is associated with happiness because it can provide a deep sense of community and support.

When we have weak social systems, many other aspects of our health are impacted. It increases our risk for loneliness and social isolation. Loneliness is not the same as social isolation. It's the feeling of being alone despite the amount of social contact. Whereas social isolation is the absence of social connections. Some people can feel lonely without being socially isolated, but socially isolated individuals experience loneliness.

Loneliness is dangerous for our mental health because it has been linked to higher rates of depression, suicide, anxiety, heart diseases, dementia, and premature death, particularly as we get older. In addition, the older we get, some people may face situations like living alone, chronic illnesses, hearing loss, or death of a family member or friend, all of which increase the risk for loneliness and social isolation. Besides vulnerable older adults, you may become lonely and socially isolated if, for instance, you migrate to a new place and have difficulties speaking the language or forming relationships with the locals.

Your social health can equally influence your self-esteem. Your social support systems serve as a safe space to find yourself, develop assertive skills, and become comfortable with yourself in social settings. It equally helps you build emotional resilience. There are a few ways you can begin to support your social health:

Join a community: Religious organizations, clubs, programs are excellent ways to get involved in your local community. Joining a community helps you meet like-minded individuals. One of the greatest benefits of joining a group is that it helps combat isolation. This is a good opportunity to meet other individuals who may also be struggling with isolation or facing similar struggles as you, and that reassurance is validating. Working for a common cause can help you feel like you belong to that community. You'll feel needed, which can give you a sense of identity. Group settings are a great way to learn from others and acquire vital information to enrich your life.

Interact more in-person: While we can still meet people virtually, in-person connections provide a different level of happiness that virtual connections don't. You can hold hands, hug, and share meals. Face-to-face interactions will always trump online connections. With in-person meetings, it's easier to study and get to know a new person on a deeper level versus only relying on what you're being told. You can speed up the conversation to learn more about the person. You can also immediately decide if you want to keep meeting them or not.

Learn to set boundaries: As you interact with people of different personalities, you'll quickly identify which bring toxic energy and which ones don't. This is where setting boundaries is crucial. A boundary is a limit or space between you and another person. Setting boundaries is good for your mental health, and it's an integral part of establishing your identity. Boundaries can be emotional or physical, and they can be rigid or loose. When you set healthy boundaries with people, you've indicated what you will and will not tolerate. Setting boundaries makes it easier to walk away from friendships and relationships that are negatively affecting your health.

4. Mental health

Our mental health refers to the ability of our brain to perform cognitive functions like reasoning, learning, making smart judgments, remembering, attention, etc. Our brain needs to be in a healthy state to perform these functions. Our mental health encompasses our social, psychological, and emotional health. This means it impacts how we feel, act, think, handle stress, and form interpersonal relationships. Mental health is vital at every stage in life. It can change over time due to factors in people. If you're burdened by demands that exceed your coping abilities, your mental health can suffer. For example, if you're working 80 hours a week without sufficient sleep, your mental health will decline. Caring for your mental health can help you live a more enjoyable life. Lifestyle choices, the genes we inherited, and socioeconomic pressures all shape a person's mental health. Any deviation from the normal functioning of our brain will result in mental health illnesses.

Mental illnesses can substantially affect all areas of a person's life, such as their ability to participate in the community, work or school performance, and interpersonal relationships. The most common mental health problems are anxiety disorders, schizophrenia, and mood disorders.

- **Anxiety disorders:** Anxiety is the most common mental illness. People with this condition have severe anxiety or fear for something or situations. Examples of anxiety disorders include:
- **Generalized anxiety disorder (GAD):** This is a condition where a person worries over everything, even when there's no reason to. This type of anxiety can disrupt everyday living. People with GAD can worry and become anxious about chores or daily activities. It can keep people from accomplishing daily responsibilities and getting through the day.

- **Panic disorders:** People with panic disorders experience unexpected panic attacks such as trembling, sweating, heart palpitations, etc. For some people, certain things trigger panic attacks, like a history of physical or sexual abuse or moving to a new home. But a person can also experience panic attacks without any triggers.
- **Phobias:** Phobia is an excessive fear of a situation or an object. People who fear spiders, ants, and bugs have a simple phobia. Sometimes the fear can be about being in social settings. This type of phobia is called social anxiety or social phobia. If you suffer from this problem, meeting new people and attending social gatherings can be challenging. A different type of phobia known as agoraphobia is a fear of being in situations where getting away may be difficult, such as being in an elevator or train.
- **Obsessive-compulsive disorder (OCD):** This anxiety disorder causes

a person to experience obsessive and compulsive urge to perform repetitive acts like cleaning the house or handwashing. Many people with OCD cannot stop the unreasonable and unnecessary repetitive thoughts.

- **Post-traumatic stress disorder (PTSD):** This illness is triggered after witnessing or experiencing a profoundly stressful or traumatic event like rape, war, or abuse of any sort where the person felt helpless or shocked.

Schizophrenia: This mental illness causes a person to have a skewed perception of the world around them. They may hear voices, hallucinate, and have delusions.

Our mental health has on our physical health is more evident in chronic illnesses. Poor mental health affects our ability to think critically and make healthy decisions. Multiple studies have noted that mental illness is closely associated with fatigue. For example, anxiety and depression often result in persistent feelings of mental exhaustion. Being mentally tired leads to physical tiredness. When someone is always physically exhausted, they're less likely to engage in exercise. Chronic physical fatigue can also interfere with your basic hygiene, increasing your vulnerability to diseases.

What's more, our mental health significantly impacts our immune system. A strong immune system keeps us away from illnesses that can negatively affect our physical bodies. For example, immune disorders like inflammatory bowel disease alter the proportion of fat mass and lean muscle mass in our bodies, affecting our bone health. Conversely, poor mental health can weaken your immune system by suppressing your immune cells, particularly your T cells, decreasing your body's ability to fight bacteria and viruses. This can make you stay sick longer.

There are ways to improve your mental health:

Cut off unhealthy lifestyles like excessive drinking, consuming recreational drugs, and smoking.

Eat foods that support your gut health. Since your gut is directly connected to your brain, a healthy gut may keep your mind healthy.

Always keep your mind active by challenging yourself and seeking out learning opportunities.

Foods that are rich in omega-3 fatty acids and antioxidants support cognitive function.

5. Spiritual health

Your spiritual health is more than belonging to a religious group. Instead, it's about connecting to a higher power. Of course, religion is one way to connect to a supernatural force that's greater than you. For some, the big question may be, "Is religion the same as spirituality?" The answer is no. They mean two different things. There are specific sets of beliefs that followers are expected to adhere to with religion. However, there may or may not be any rules or a particular belief system in spirituality. It's just a feeling people get regarding something greater than them. It's possible to be religious and spiritual simultaneously or to be spiritual yet not religious. It all boils down to your motive for choosing either one of them.

Religion often involves believing in supernatural powers like Buddha, God, or Allah. You may find that actively engaging with your belief regularly strengthens your faith if you're religious. Practices like praying, joining a group with other like minds, and regularly going to your place of worship can help you find meaning in religion. In turn, you'll feel a greater sense of purpose in life.

Religion serves many purposes in our lives. People turn to religion for comfort and guidance. It can provide a moral compass to help people regulate their behaviours, develop healthy habits, and better understand their emotions, positively impacting their health. Specific religions may encourage healthy behaviours. For example, the Mormons or Seventh Day Adventists live a lifestyle of no alcohol, tobacco, or drug use. Instead, they consume more whole grains, fruits, and vegetables, reduce their meat intake, and engage in more physical activity. Belonging to a religion provides a sense of community and connection to others and a higher entity, beneficial for your health.

If you're not religious, spending time in nature can make you feel connected to a greater power. Nature is made up of both living and nonliving things. Nature's living things include plants and animals, while nonliving things consist of water, rocks, and other lifeless things. Humans have always explored nature to derive food, medicinal substances, shelter, or clothing. The sounds of wildlife, the cool atmospheric temperature created by large canopy trees, and the rustling of leaves can positively affect your overall health.

THERE ARE different ways of connecting with nature. You can connect with nature by physically interacting with it. This is as simple as spending time in green spaces around you or visiting your local park. Besides seeing nature, you can connect with nature by hearing, touching, and smelling nature. Our emotions and our sense of smell are connected. The smell of a house plant, for instance, might make us feel happier and calmer. You can equally build a relationship with nature by listening to the sounds of flowing water or cricket chirping. As you spend more time in nature, you'll begin to form a deeper connection with your environment. You'll feel more emotionally and psychologically connected with the natural world.

Caring for your spiritual health is just as important as caring for other aspects of your health. Our spiritual health often becomes more important in times of emotional stress or illness. When we're spiritually healthy, we feel connected to a higher power and others around us. We have more clarity with our choices, and whatever we do will be in line with our beliefs and values.

Someone spiritually healthy knows their purpose in life and can reflect on the meaning of events. They know what is right and wrong, which guides their actions. A spiritually healthy person displays hope, self-acceptance or forgiveness, clear values, a positive outlook, self-worth, and a sense of peace, which is good for your mental and emotional health. In comparison, a spiritually unhealthy person may experience a lack of meaning in life, apathy, feelings of emptiness, self-judgment, anxiety, and conflicting values.

If you think you need to improve your spiritual health, here are some ways to do it:

- Pray regularly—in a group or alone.

- Spend more time in nature.
- Practice yoga and meditation.
- Read and listen to inspirational materials.
- Get involved in your community.
- Self-reflect and find what makes you feel happy, loved, peaceful, and connected.

STEPS TOWARD HOLISTIC HEALTH AND NUTRITION

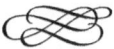

Science tells us that it can be challenging to change our lifestyle all at once. So instead, we should start with a few things we want to alter and work from there. For instance, If you want to change your eating habit to a healthier one or start an exercise routine, begin to take sustainable and straightforward steps at a time. More minor changes are easier to achieve, and the feeling of success you get can motivate you to continue to make lifestyle changes.

An old adage says it takes 21 days to form a habit. However, this may or may not be accurate for everyone. Some people may need more than 21 days. So when you begin to make minor changes, don't be too hard on yourself if the new changes don't stick right away. It can take a while before a new behaviour becomes second nature. Some tasks are quicker to learn than others.

GUIDE to Holistic Health

If you're interested in starting your journey through holistic health with nutrition, here are some fundamental steps to follow. As always, consult your doctor before making any changes to your lifestyle, especially if you're taking prescription medications.

- **STEP 1:** Good health starts in the kitchen! The cure for most of our illnesses can be found in the kitchen. It's a place to nourish our bodies and souls and try new recipes. We've been led to believe that cooking healthy foods is time-consuming and expensive. Hence, we rely on already made foods, which are deemed inexpensive. But these foods can cause illnesses that cost hundreds of dollars per month.

HOLISTIC HEALTH AND NUTRITION

What we put in our bodies is essential to living a life of wellness. And a sure way to be in complete control of your nutrition is to prepare your own meals. By preparing your own meal, you know what was added and the amounts. That way, you can control for each ingredient. For example, you can decrease your salt intake or increase your protein intake depending on your dietary needs. So begin by stocking your fridge with more fresh fruits and vegetables and remove all prepackaged, processed, and sugary foods. If you don't know where to buy whole foods, look for any whole food store around you or the best farmer's market. By consuming a healthy diet, you're caring for all dimensions of your well-being.

The types of foods we eat allow our bodies to work at the fullest potential. They play a vital role in how we feel emotionally, mentally, and physically. If you eat more whole foods, your cells and organs will be energized by the nutrients they provide, and you'll feel better overall. This is key to keeping you healthy.

- **STEP 2:** Determine why you bought

this book and what bothers you about your health and wellness. Everything happens for a reason. I'm sure you had particular reasons for purchasing this book and what you hope to learn from it. It'll be difficult to get much out of anything if you don't have a purpose or reason for doing it in the first place. If your reason is related to your overall health and well-being, what about it do you want to change? These are questions you must ask yourself before you start altering any aspect of your lifestyle.

The aim of outlining your reasons is to help you make logical decisions about how you want to accomplish your goals. By the end of this book, set goals of what you would like to achieve with your overall health and well-being; for example, your goal may be to get rid of bloating, headaches, or fatigue.

After setting goals, plan the steps you must take to actualize each one and cross off the points you've accomplished. This will motivate you and help you focus your mindset on each idea on your to-do list. Without goals, you'll lack focus and direction, and you won't have a tool to evaluate your success. One of my favourite ways to set goals is to use the acronym "SMART," which stands for:

S—specific
M—measurable
A—attainable
R—relevant
T—trackable

- **STEP 3**: Start a journal of what you eat, when you eat, and how you feel after you eat.

Journaling helps you keep track of your intentions to achieve your goals. You'll be able to see how much progress you have made and remind yourself of what you need to do to accomplish the remaining goals.

Begin journaling by recording what you've eaten and what you're eating. Record how you felt mentally, physically, and emotionally after eating each food. After a week or two, go back to your journal and see any patterns and trends. You'll be able to understand your eating habits and sensitivities. Determine whether the food you ate gave you any discomfort. Did you feel bloated or tired after eating certain foods? If so, eliminate that food from your diet. And move to the next step to help you determine foods that aid your body, not harm it. Are there any foods you ate that made you feel energetic?

Take your findings into consideration when shopping for your next meal. If you're unsure of your results or think there may be other confounding factors that may have influenced how you felt, try eliminating those foods from your diet for a week and observe how your body responds to them. It might take some time to figure out which foods are best for your health and which ones aren't. Food journaling is one of the most effective methods of ensuring you're eating more whole foods and reducing your intake of unhealthy ones.

- **STEP 4:** Apply the 80/20 rule. The idea behind the 80/20 rule for your diet is to make sure you're eating whole, unprocessed foods 80% of the time, while the remaining 20% can be for less healthy foods.

HOLISTIC HEALTH AND NUTRITION

It's nearly impossible to eat healthy foods 100% of the time. Life happens, and you can't always control everything. You might be at a place where processed foods are the only food items available, or it's that time of the year to celebrate, and pastries are the only foods provided. What do you do then? It isn't sustainable long-term to deprive yourself of the foods you once loved before you began eating healthy. It's ok to have your favourite desserts from time to time, provided you don't binge eat. The 80/20 rule aims to help you create a balanced and healthy life without feeling guilty after consuming less healthy foods. In addition, it prevents you from developing an unhealthy relationship with food.

What healthy foods can you eat 80% of the time? Fruits and vegetables, whole grains, legumes and beans, healthy fats, and lots of fluids, especially water. You can still eat meat and dairy, but if you aren't vegan or vegetarian, reduce their intake to decrease the amount of saturated fat in your diet. And when purchasing meat or dairy, always buy grass-fed, organic, and free-range options, as they're leaner and lower in calories than other options. That said, your focus while applying this rule should center on foods that will improve your overall well-being. Even while you indulge 20% of the time, eat only high-quality foods.

- **STEP 5**: Practice intuitive eating. Intuitive eating is all about nourishing your body in a sustainable way, whereby there's no restriction on what you can and cannot eat. It's not a diet; it's a way of life. If anything, eating intuitively safeguards you from falling into the diet culture. It allows you to focus on what's most important for your well-being.

Sometimes additional constraints can impact our food choices. For example, you might not have time to regularly prepare fresh foods or shop for organic foods in bulk. Or you might be living on a budget and can't spend a fortune on food. However, you can still nourish your body if you focus on consuming nutrient-dense foods rather than foods others define as healthy. With intuitive eating, only do what works for you, your lifestyle, and your budget. For instance, you can buy frozen fruits and vegetables if you can't always afford fresh ones. Fortified cereals are also rich in micronutrients.

As you practice intuitive eating, be mindful of what you eat, when you eat it, why you're eating it, and how you feel after consuming certain foods. Here are some tips to master mindfulness during meals:

1. Eat your meals slowly to allow your body time to digest. If possible, place your fork down between each bite.
2. Every morning, squeeze half of a whole lemon into a glass of water and drink. Before and after every meal, also drink a glass of water. But avoid consuming too much liquid during meals. Instead, take small sips in between.
3. Eat with no distractions.
4. Eat home-cooked foods so you know what you are eating.

- **STEP 6:** Take one day at a time and do not stress if you choose to eat something that your body doesn't agree with. Learn to live for the moment and enjoy every hour that goes by. As much as possible, avoid overthinking about your food choices. It's ok if one of your meals wasn't healthy, as long as it doesn't become a habit. Don't obsess over your food's nutritional quality to the degree that it can damage your overall well-being and become an eating disorder. Instead, acknowledge that you made that food choice, understand how it made you feel, and move on.

Continue to live a healthy lifestyle and eat nutritious foods. Your body will get used to healthy foods and crave more of them in time. Our taste buds crave what we feed them. Why don't we crave salad the same way we crave cheeseburgers? It's because we've conditioned ourselves to want these unhealthy foods. If you regularly consume sugary foods, your taste buds will crave more of them, causing you to gravitate more toward sugary foods like desserts, pop drinks, cookies, etc. But you can retrain your taste buds to want healthy foods. For example, the more you eat those bitter vegetables that you initially didn't like, they'll begin to taste better to you over time.

- **STEP 7:** At this point, you should have a better understanding of what foods your body does not agree with. You should know what foods make you feel energized and which ones don't. Moreover, you should now have a better understanding of why you gravitate toward certain foods and not others, your eating habits, and how to make healthy food choices.

This is when you should begin cutting out toxic foods from your diet. In addition, any food that doesn't enrich your health should be removed. This includes foods that are high in calories but nutrient-poor.

There are painless ways to do it:

1. If you eat a significant amount of processed foods, slowly remove them from your diet. You might not

be able to cut off all processed foods at once, but the slower you ease into less-processed foods, the more you're likely to continue in your healthy lifestyle.
2. Plan your meals if necessary. If you reach for unhealthy foods because of convenience, try preparing your foods ahead. You may need to package some fresh fruits, yogurts, and other healthier snacks that are ready to grab and go.
3. Pick healthier alternatives. Instead of potato chips, try plain popcorn. Water or freshly squeezed juices are a better alternative to pop. You can equally replace sweetened cereals for unsweetened oatmeal topped with fruits . Likewise, you can improve the flavour of your food by sprinkling garlic or black pepper in place of extra salt. You can supplement your breakfast snacks with fresh fruits and vegetables like bananas or apples for breakfast.

After eliminating all unhealthy and

processed foods from your diet, stick to wholesome foods and stay away from processed and packaged foods.

- **STEP 8:** Combine healthy foods the proper way to improve your gut health. Don't normalize feeling bloated or producing excessive gas after a meal. It's your body's way of telling you something is wrong. If you aren't sure how to combine your foods, go to chapter three of this book, where I explained it in detail. You can equally do a quick internet search. Or simply listen to your body during and after every meal and write down the effects they have on your body. By observing patterns from your meals, you'll know which ones are better for your gut.

- **STEP 9:** Alkalize your body. I elaborated on this nutritional concept in chapter three. It's easy! Eat more whole foods, reduce/eliminate unhealthy foods from your diet, and reduce your intake of animal protein sources. Not only will it protect you from diseases, but your body will also be nourished.

Besides your diet, exercise helps restore your body's pH to a healthy range. Aerobic exercises are especially beneficial to balance your body's pH because it helps to reduce the accumulation of acid in your body. Make sure to do at least one form of exercise every day, whether it's walking, running, gardening, or swimming.

- **STEP 10:** Exercise – be active daily, even if all you do is go for a walk. Regular exercise is good for your overall health. It's an excellent weight loss strategy a good stress management technique, and it lowers your risk for certain chronic illnesses.

You can start exercising with these few tips:

HOLISTIC HEALTH AND NUTRITION

1. Make it part of your routine. There's no set day and time to exercise. The best time to exercise is one that fits into your lifestyle. So schedule days and times of the week to get in at least 30 minutes of exercise. This will help you stick to your workout routine. I recommend exercising in the morning to avoid distractions from your other daily obligations. However, any time of the day is equally good.
2. Be part of an exercise group or bring a friend.
3. Incorporate resistance exercises. Try to do some strength training exercises twice a week to build your muscle mass and strengthen your bones. This will boost your metabolism as well. You can begin with lighter weights or use your body weight for exercises like push-ups, pull-ups, sit-ups, lunges, and squats to strengthen your body.

- **STEP 11:** Incorporate psycho-spiritual therapy into your lifestyle.

This is where you first break down the five aspects of holistic health to see how they relate to you, then integrate psycho-spiritual methods to areas that require work to achieve optimal health.

Psycho-spiritual therapy is a practice that integrates both psychological and spiritual methods (such as meditation, yoga, dreamwork, and breathwork) in a holistic, integrated approach. It recognizes that our psychological and spiritual development are inseparable, and our spiritual health influences our psychic health and overall development. This holistic approach to health assumes that our psychological development is an essential component of our spiritual growth. It incorporates the mind, body, and soul, which results in a deeper level of health, understanding and awareness of yourself, and unconditional love for yourself. So if you feel hopeless or feel like you've lost a part of yourself, psycho-spiritual therapy may be something for you to consider.

I will go over a few psycho-spiritual

methods to help you find ways to allow your body to relax from your day-to-day stresses.

- **Music therapy:** Music can improve your overall well-being.

It can reflect different emotions. Songs can indirectly express what we're feeling without us verbalizing it. You can perform various activities during music therapy like writing songs, playing an instrument, listening to different melodies, and guided imagery. And it's appropriate for people of any age and health condition whether you're healthy or not.

This form of therapy impacts our mind, body, and brain by distracting our mind from personal problems, relaxing our bodies, and improving our mood. It awakens a deeper level of emotional experience and awareness. So you may experience a feeling of moving beyond your current situation into a broader psycho-spiritual realm.

- **Massage:** This practice is typically done by a certified professional. The therapist uses different degrees of pressure and movement to manipulate the soft tissues of your body, such as your tendons, muscle, joints, ligaments, and connective tissue. Massage is beneficial to our overall health. It can help you relax, lessen muscle tension and pain, and reduce stress. You can use this practice to treat various health conditions, from acute to chronic illnesses. And it's safe for all age groups.

- **Dream-work**: Our dreams are unique and may convey what we're thinking about, our emotions, concerns, and memories. Dream therapy requires you to make a note of your dream each morning and bring it with you to therapy. Your therapist will then guide you through it to help you discover the meaning. But your therapist will not interpret or analyze your dream. The more you carry out this practice, the better you understand yourself, improving your well-being.

- **Meditation**: This involves a set of techniques that increase your focus and attention and allows you to be present in the moment.

Meditation has been practiced in numerous cultures and traditions worldwide for thousands of years. In addition, nearly all religious denominations involve a few meditation techniques in their practice.

There are nine different meditation techniques: focused meditation, spiritual meditation, mindfulness meditation, movement meditation, loving-kindness meditation, mantra meditation, transcendental meditation, progressive relaxation, and visualization meditation.

- **Acupuncture:** This practice requires a practitioner to insert tiny needles through your skin at strategic points on your body.

The scientific basis of how acupuncture functions are still unclear. However, it is believed that acupuncture points are places on your body that can stimulate your nerves, connective tissue, and muscle. Once they become stimulated, they increase blood flow throughout the body while at the same time triggering the release of the body's natural painkillers.

Traditional Chinese medicine believes it'll increase energy flow throughout your body by applying acupuncture, thereby improving your health. In the practice of acupuncture, it's believed that illnesses are caused by an imbalance of energy flow in our bodies. So applying acupuncture will restabilize the energy flow. This practice is commonly used to reduce pain, but it can also manage stress and improve your overall well-being.

SUPPLEMENTS AND NUTRITION COMBINED

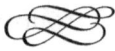

Dietary supplements are an excellent addition to a healthy lifestyle. Supplements are rich in vitamins, minerals, enzymes, amino acids, herbs and other botanicals, and many other good ingredients for your body. They can provide adequate amounts of essential nutrients lacking in your diet if you don't eat nutritious foods. But supplements shouldn't take the place of a healthy diet. They can't provide all the benefits that whole foods, fruits, and vegetables provide. Whole foods provide essential fibre, a wide variety of micronutrients that your body needs, and they are rich in antioxidants.

Who needs supplements? You don't need supplements if you eat a wide variety of foods such as fruits, low-fat dairy products, lean meats, whole grains, vegetables, fish, and legumes. However, supplements may be appropriate if you're pregnant or trying to, above the age of 50, follow a restrictive diet that excludes certain food groups, have an illness that affects how your body digests nutrients, or you have a poor appetite.

There are dietary supplements for different nutritional needs and come in various forms: such as pills, powders, drinks, tablets, energy bars, and gummies. The most popular ones are vitamins B12, D, probiotics, fish oil, iron, calcium, glucosamine, and herbs such as garlic and echinacea.

Every supplement comes with a label that lists the active ingredients, doses, and other substances used to manufacture the supplement. Typically, the manufacturer suggests the serving size, but consult your doctor before proceeding. They might decide a different amount is more appropriate for you.

When you begin to add supplements to your diet, you may have side effects from some of them. This is because the active ingredients present can substantially impact our bodies. In addition, side effects are bound to occur if you take supplements at high doses or consume too many supplements. So always be alert to the possibility of a bad reaction.

Role of Supplements in Holistic Nutritional Health

Supplementing your diet may contribute to the wellness objective of helping your body, mind, and spirit. Dietary supplements are essential for your overall well-being for the following reasons:

- **It maintains your general health.** Our bodies need vitamins A, C, D, E, and K, and B vitamins such as folate/folic acid, riboflavin (B2), thiamin (B1), pantothenic acid (B5), niacin (B3), cobalamin (B12), biotin, and pyridoxal (B6). The minerals essential for health are calcium, phosphorus, potassium, sodium, chloride, magnesium, iron, zinc, iodine, sulphur, cobalt, copper, fluoride, manganese, and selenium.

Multivitamins provide these 28 micronutrients in the right amounts required for optimal health, so supplementing your diet is a great way to meet your recommended daily allowance of these micronutrients.

Each micronutrient plays a specific role in our bodies. Many of these micronutrients are essential in producing hormones and enzymes. Some boost our immunity to protect against illnesses. Our bodies require some to support the functioning of our nerves and organs and to maintain these structures. In addition, these essential micronutrients play a crucial role in our bodies during reproduction, growth, maintenance, and regulation of physiological processes.

For instance, our bodies need calcium and vitamin D to strengthen our bones and reduce bone loss. Vitamin D also helps keep our colon healthy and prevent colon cancer. It's been proven that folic acid can decrease the risk of congenital disabilities and may reduce the risk of colon cancer, heart disease, breast cancer, and other types of cancer. B vitamins are known for their ability to increase our energy and support the functioning of our nervous system. Magnesium might help relax our bodies. The omega-3 fatty acids in fish oils might help keep your heart healthy.

Numerous studies have shown that antioxidants can help prevent certain cancers. In addition, nutrients like vitamin C and Zinc are proven to boost our immune system. What's more, the combination of fat-soluble antioxidants such as lutein and zeaxanthin together with vitamins C, E, zinc, and copper may protect your eyes and slow down vision loss as you age. These are just a few health benefits that supplements have to offer.

- **It helps prevent nutritional deficiencies.** When our bodies are not getting enough nutrients in the right amounts, we can become deficient in nutrients. The first evidence of nutrient deficiency was observed in 1747 among sailors sick with scurvy. To ascertain the cure for the illness, all the sailors were split into different groups, consuming other natural remedies such as garlic, lemon, orange, mustard, and garlic. However, only the sailors who consumed citrus fruits recovered. So it was noted that vitamin C was the limiting nutrient and the only nutrient that can protect us from scurvy. After this discovery, other micronutrients emerged associated with specific disease states.

Globally, nutrient deficiency is still a problem. The micronutrients of most concern are folate, vitamin A, zinc, iron, vitamin D, and iodine. Vitamin A deficiency, for instance, is most prevalent in developing countries. However, developed countries may have more problems with vitamin D deficiency, especially in cold countries with insufficient sunlight exposure for several months of the year.

When you're deficient in micronutrients, your body uses signs and symptoms to communicate this problem to you.

Here are the most common symptoms you may experience:

- **Skin problems:** Disorders like dandruff and seborrheic dermatitis (SB) are common with a poor nutrient diet. They typically affect areas of your body that produce oil. Both conditions cause itchy, flaking skin. SB mostly appears on the armpit, upper chest, groin, and face, while dandruff is restricted to the scalp. With dandruff, flakes of the skin can range from small and white flakes to large, greasy, and yellow flakes. SB causes redness on a light skin tone and light patches on a darker skin tone.

Low levels of nutrients like zinc, niacin, riboflavin, and pyridoxine may be responsible for these skin problems since they play a role in our skin health and maintenance. In addition, the likelihood of developing these skin disorders is highest during the first three months of life, during puberty, and in mid-adulthood.

By consuming foods rich in these nutrients, you may be protecting yourself against these skin problems. Niacin, riboflavin, and pyridoxine can be found in whole foods, dairy, meat, and fish. In addition, whole grains, seafood, meat, nuts, and seeds are excellent sources of zinc.

- **Bleeding gums.** Your gums can bleed from either brushing your teeth too hard or not getting sufficient micronutrients from your diet, particularly vitamin C.

Increased bleeding is one of the symptoms of scurvy, which affected sailors without access to fruits and vegetables.

Fruits and vegetables are very high in vitamin C. So you can be deficient in this nutrient if you don't consume enough fruits and vegetables. Vitamin C is crucial in preventing periodontal diseases.

Besides bleeding gums, other symptoms of vitamin C deficiency include weak muscles and bones, low immunity, fatigue and lethargy, slow wound healing, tooth loss, and frequent nose bleeds.

In supplements, vitamin C comes in the form of ascorbic acid.

- **Hair loss:** This is when your hair isn't growing, and no new hair replaces your lost hair. Anybody can lose their hair. It can be hereditary, caused by hormonal changes, caused by tight hairstyles, or caused by a lack of certain nutrients. It's normal to lose your hair the older you get. However, the following nutrients are essential for healthy hair:
- Zinc: Our hair is made up of a protein called keratin. Zinc is essential to synthesize new keratin for hair growth. Any zinc deficiency can cause hair loss. As such, you should increase your intake of zinc.
- Iron: This nutrient, just like zinc, is required for hair growth. It is needed to synthesize new DNA molecules present in our hair follicles. Without sufficient iron intake, our hair can fall out or stop growing.
- Biotin: This B-vitamin stimulates the keratin production in hair and regrows lost hair.

- Niacin: This B-vitamin helps to increase blood circulation to our hair follicles, which is necessary for a healthy scalp. That's right! Poor blood circulation can cause your hair to fall out in small patches, a condition known as alopecia.
- Essential fatty acids: We need fatty acids like Linoleic acid (LA) and alpha-linolenic acid (ALA) for hair growth and maintenance. ALA is a plant-based omega-3 fatty acid found in nuts like flaxseed oil, canola, and walnut oils. In comparison, LA is an omega-6 fatty acid found in vegetable oils, nuts, seeds, and animal products. However, you can still get these nutrients from supplements.

If you're already getting these nutrients from your diet, there's no need to take vitamin and mineral supplements as it may worsen your hair loss rather than help it.

- **Vision problems:** Nutrient deficiency, particularly vitamin A, can cause you to have poor vision in low light or darkness or cause white growths on your eyes. We need vitamin A for healthy vision, healthy skin, fetal growth and development, and the normal functioning of our immune system. Vitamin A is necessary to produce a pigment called rhodopsin found in the retina of our eyes. It's this pigment that allows us to see at night. Poor vision at night (night blindness) may not affect your normal vision in the daytime.

Night blindness is a preventable condition that can be reversed with a sufficient intake of vitamin A. However, when left untreated, night blindness can progress into xerophthalmia, a condition that can damage your vision and lead to permanent blindness.

Vitamin A deficiency can also show up as foamy, white spots on the white part of your eyes. The white spots are keratin build-up. They can be oval, triangular, or irregular in shape. You equally need to consume sufficient vitamin A to eliminate the white spots.

Most developed countries rarely have a vitamin A deficiency problem. So unless diagnosed with a deficiency, avoid taking vitamin A supplements because excess vitamin A in the body is toxic.

- **Small bumps on the skin**: The appearance of goosebump-like bumps on the skin may be due to inadequate intake of vitamins A and C. These bumps are painless and are usually your skin colour. They can appear red on white skin and brownish-black on dark skin. They can appear on the thighs, cheeks, buttocks, arms. Some can have ingrown or corkscrew hairs.

This condition is known as Keratosis pilaris. It can affect people of any age, but it often appears in childhood and naturally disappears in adulthood. Keratosis pilaris may appear when too much keratin is produced in hair follicles. Nobody is still 100% sure why it builds up, but there may be a genetic component to it, meaning if your parents have it, you may get it too.

Thus, supplements can help fill nutritional gaps in your diet and protect you against these health problems.

- **It supports sports-related performance.** An athlete's nutrition can make a difference in their performance. Some athletes need to supplement their diet, while others don't if they eat a balanced diet. For instance, if an athlete is vegan, they may have to take supplements for other nutrients lacking in their diet. Proper nutrition is vital in sports because it provides the energy to perform high-intensity exercises.

Nutritional supplementation has always been something that helps athletes quickly recover between training sessions and reduce training interruptions due to illnesses. There are different types of sports supplements, each performing a unique function. They include energy bars, sports drinks, protein supplements, and meal replacements. However, there is evidence that supplements like creatine, caffeine, bicarbonate, and others can improve sports performance.

Creatine is frequently used by athletes in track and field sports since there are no harmful effects, even in high doses. The highest amount of creatine is found in the skeletal muscles in our bodies. Creatine helps to generate energy for our cells. By taking a creatine supplement, you're increasing muscle creatine, thereby increasing how much energy is produced to support your high-intensity activities.

Caffeine is a popular substance that's found in many foods and beverages. If you're a coffee drinker, you should be familiar with this word. Caffeine improves sports performance in so many ways. It positively affects our central nervous system by increasing our ability to focus during performance. It also has effects on our skeletal muscles and our fat cells. Caffeine may increase the breakdown of fat from fat cells to generate more energy.

Other supplements like sodium bicarbonate may enhance your sports performance by reducing lactic acid build-up in your muscles. During an intense exercise, lactic acid is produced within our muscles.

However, too much of it can build up and cause burning sensations in your muscles.

Effects of Nutrition and Supplement on Our Brain

Our brain health is just as important as the health of other cells and organs in our bodies. A healthy brain can perform all cognitive processes such as thinking, memory, perception, and creation of imagery. However, as we age, our brains undergo structural changes. These changes included a loss of gray matter in the brain and a decrease in the size of brain areas. And these changes impact our cognitive abilities.

The gray matter is the outermost layer of our brain. It plays a vital role in healthy cognitive functioning. It contains the highest concentration of neurons and brain cells. Each neuron is responsible for a different brain function. So the nerves that control different cognitive abilities like learning and memory, thinking, perception, regulating our emotions, and creating imagery are all located in the gray matter. Therefore, an age-related decrease in the amount of gray matter in our brain can lead to cognitive decline.

The hippocampus and cerebellum are

regions of our brain that regulate different brain functions. The hippocampus controls our cognitive abilities like learning and memory. It's also the part of our brain that increases in size as more neurons are produced in the brain. And the more neurons are made, the stronger the connection between different brain regions and the better our brain can coordinate other functions. Like the hippocampus, the cerebellum is responsible for our cognitive abilities like language and attention. It's equally involved in coordinating our movement and balance.

To keep your brain healthy, nutritional supplementation has been shown to impact cognition positively by implementing supplements like fruits, teas, spices, vitamins, folate, and fish oil in your diet.

Fish oil contains omega-3 fatty acids. This type of fat is an essential structural component of every organ and structure we have in our body, even our brain. There are different types of omega-3 fatty acids available, but the one that's of most importance to our brain is docosahexaenoic acid (DHA). DHA makes up approximately 90% of the omega-3 fatty acid in our brain. It is the building block of all our brain cells. This fat binds to the cell membrane of each brain cell, increasing its fluidity. This makes it easier for nerve cells to communicate with one another. When the levels of DHA in our brain become low, it can alter the functioning of our brain.

Our bodies cannot produce enough DHA, so you must get it from your diet or take supplements. DHA is critical for healthy brain aging. As we age, not only does the size and weight of our brain decrease, but the fat content decreases as well. So taking a DHA supplement may improve the cognitive functioning of our brain, especially in those with mild memory loss.

Accumulated evidence for other supplements like selenium has also been shown to improve the cognitive functioning of an aging brain. Selenium is important for cognition by reducing oxidative stress in the body. Accumulation of free radicals is very toxic to our bodies, especially our brains since its composition and physiology make it more susceptible. Our brain requires lots of oxygen to function well. High amounts of free radicals are generated during their oxygen consumption relative to other organs in our bodies. If free radicals accumulate, they can damage the neurons in our brain.

Selenium deficiency places our brains at higher risk for oxidative stress damage, leading to cognitive decline and altered brain function. So consuming foods rich in selenium is one of the best ways to protect your brain from oxidative stress. You can get adequate selenium from protein-rich foods like fish, meat, and legumes. Taking a selenium supplement is equally beneficial but only for dietary restrictions that exclude these protein-rich foods.

Examples of Holistic Health Supplements

There are seven crucial supplements for your holistic health. They include:

- **Vitamin D3**: Vitamin D is essential for healthy skin, a stronger immune system, and a happier mood. For most people, it isn't easy to get the required amount of this nutrient from the diet, so it's best to take a supplement. Vitamin D supplement comes in two forms: vitamin D2 and vitamin D3. Vitamin D3 comes naturally from the sun's ultraviolet-

B (UVB) rays, hence its nickname, "the sunshine vitamin." I mentioned earlier that your climate could affect how much vitamin D3 you get. So if you're regularly exposed to sunlight, there's no need to take a supplement.

Since the sun produces high amounts of UVB rays between 10 am and 2 pm, this is the best time to get this nutrient. If you're unsure how much vitamin D3 you're getting, do a test to see whether you're deficient. But you most certainly are if you aren't regularly exposed to the sun.

- **Iodine:** Iodine is an important component of the thyroid hormones thyroxine (T4) and triiodothyronine (T3). These hormones regulate our metabolism and many important biological processes in our bodies. When there's sufficient iodine in your diet, the thyroid gland will be able to use the iodine to produce T4 and T3. Without adequate iodine, these hormones won't be produced, and a condition known as goiter can arise.

Iodine is one of those nutrients that most people are deficient in. In the United States, approximately 96% of the population doesn't get enough iodine from their diet. This is due to substances like bromine and pesticides; that can interfere with the uptake of iodine by the thyroid gland. Numerous studies have linked insufficient iodine intake to chronic fatigue, depression, and fibromyalgia. Fortunately, iodine is available as sodium iodide or potassium iodide supplement.

- **Omega-3 fatty acid:** Like iodine, 90% of the United States population aren't getting enough omega-3 fatty acid in their diet. Dietary supplements will be beneficial if you aren't eating foods rich in this nutrient, either from plant or animal sources.
- **Probiotics**: Probiotics are those beneficial bacteria that keep our gut healthy. They help balance the "good" and "bad" bacteria in your

gut. They equally help our bodies absorb nutrients and destroy bad bacteria. Probiotics can be depleted by harmful behaviours like inadequate sleep, sugary foods, smoking, medication, and lack of exercise.

If you're having problems with your digestive system, you can take probiotic supplements. These supplements are generally considered safe since probiotics naturally exist in our bodies. However, not everyone should take a probiotic supplement, especially if you have a weakened immune system. Talk to your healthcare provider before starting a probiotic supplement.

Probiotics should not be confused with prebiotics. Prebiotics are dietary fibres that the good bacteria in your gut feed on. There are two common types of probiotic bacteria: *Bifidobacteria* and *Lactobacillus*. Other kinds include *Bacillus, Escherichia, Streptococcus, Saccharomyces,* and *Enterococcus.* Each probiotic has been found to address a unique health condition. So choosing the right type of supplement is essential. Some supplements combine different kinds of probiotics. These supplements are known as multi-probiotics or broad-spectrum probiotics.

- **Multivitamin:** It's worth taking a multivitamin if you want to protect your health. This supplement contains all the essential vitamins that your body requires. But bear in mind that even though you're taking a multivitamin supplement, you still must pay attention to your diet. It's also important to remember not to overdose on any vitamin or consume it in excess, as specific vitamins may lead to health issues. Likewise, don't consume foods that are very high in a particular vitamin in addition to your multivitamin to avoid health problems.
- **Glutathione:** This is an antioxidant produced in the liver. It consists of three amino acids— cysteine, glycine, and glutamic acid. Glutathione plays a crucial role in our bodies. It protects our cells and organs from free radicals. It equally

detoxifies our blood from harmful substances and facilitates the transport of toxins like mercury out of our cells and brains. Other functions of glutathione are repairing damaged tissues and producing beneficial chemicals and compounds. Due to its importance in our bodies, we need to maintain glutathione at a high level.

Your glutathione levels can deplete due to age, poor diet, or exposure to toxins like mercury from vaccinations, glyphosate, and other toxic substances. If your blood glutathione level is low, it's possible to increase it through supplementation. Supplements will stimulate your body to produce more glutathione naturally. Or you can turn to sulfur-rich foods like cabbage, bok choy, and kale to boost its production.

Supplements like grass-fed whey protein concentrate contain high amounts of cysteine. Cysteine is a critical precursor of glutathione synthesis. Other over-the-counter glutathione supplements are equally beneficial. If you choose to take supplements, select the liposomal form of glutathione. Liposomes can encapsulate an active ingredient, in this case, glutathione, and cross over barriers in the blood without going through the process of being destroyed by the digestive system. Because of this, its delivery into the body is more efficient than its other counterparts.

- **Multimineral:** Like multivitamins, multiminerals are supplements that contain all the essential minerals your body requires in the right amount. They're often combined with multivitamins to generate greater health benefits than when consumed separately.

AFTERWORD

Our bodies are so complex that caring for our health requires us to take a different approach than just treating the symptoms. A unique approach aims to help your whole body from the inside out. As much as possible, you should take a holistic stance when addressing issues that may arise in your life, as this is a much better and more sustainable way to a happier, healthier, and more nutritious life.

As your body begins to feel better, adopt a healthy diet consisting of whole, unprocessed foods together with lean meat, fish, and low-fat dairy products as your first step to achieving total health and wellness. The foods we eat provide the fuel and resources our bodies use to keep us healthy.

The good thing about holistic health with nutrition is personalizing it to suit your lifestyle. Since our bodies are different, we all have different needs. Therefore, your body may need more of a particular nutrient due to your lifestyle. In that case, it's advisable to take supplements to fill those nutritional gaps. However, unless your healthcare provider confirms your nutrient deficiency, it's best to stick with consuming whole, unprocessed foods rather than chugging down supplements as it may cause more harm than good.

It Starts With You!

Your health is in your hands, and only you have the power to determine what direction it goes. As the driver of your own life, you make the ultimate decision of situations that concern you. You decide whether or not you want to keep spending thousands of dollars on pharmaceutical drugs or whether you want to embark on a lifestyle that'd keep illnesses at bay.

No matter how minor something is, so far, it concerns your health; you must pay close attention to it. Those little things we neglect now may begin to haunt us the older we get. Just because you've survived on four hours of sleep for five years without any problem doesn't mean it isn't affecting other aspects of your life. Your mental health or your emotional health may be suffering. It may equally be the cause of your large appetite or your fluctuating mood.

Now that you have all the tools to live a nutritious life go out there and use them. As you begin your journey to optimal health, take one step at a time. If you stumble along the way or need guidance, you can always refer to this book. I hope that you find your pathway to total health enjoyable and stress-free.

If you have enjoyed Holistic Health and Nutrition, A Simple 11 Step Approach to Holistic Health with Nutrition, I would be very grateful if you could write a review on Amazon.com.

References

Alessi, G. (2017). The Importance of Nutritional Supplements. Balanced Well-Being Healthcare. https://www.balancedwell-

AFTERWORD

beinghealthcare.com/the-importance-of-nutritional-supplements/

American Psychological Association. (2018). Stress effects on the body. https://www.apa.org/topics/stress/body

Anderson, S. (2018). Body Systems & Nutrition. Healthfully. https://healthfully.com/body-systems-nutrition-6945663.html

Banks, C. (2018). Happiness. From Unsplash License. [Image]. https://unsplash.com/photos/POzx_amnWJw

Barboza, F. (2021). Journaling. From Unsplash License. [Image]. https://unsplash.com/photos/Lf3S2zRXKXk

Better Health Channel. (2018). Physical activity - it's important. Vic.gov.au. https://www.betterhealth.vic.gov.au/health/healthyliving/physical-activity-its-important

Bewakoof.com Official. (2017). Healthy Life. From Unsplash License. [Image]. https://unsplash.com/photos/mtOM-SpOWxRI

Brady, D. M. (2018). The Importance of Stress Reduction in Overall Health. Institute for Natural Medicine. https://naturemed.org/the-importance-of-stress-reduction-in-overall-health/

Cajina, I. (2018). Laughing. From Unsplash License. [Image]. https://unsplash.com/photos/dnL6ZIpht2s

Carter, L. (2021). What is the Gut-Brain Axis? | Spencer Institute. Spencer Institute Coach Certification & Business Training. https://spencerinstitute.com/gut-brain-axis/

Chesak, J. (2018). The No-BS Guide to Holistic, Healthier Eating. Healthline. https://www.healthline.com/health/food-nutrition/how-to-start-intuitive-eating

Cottonbro. (2020). Stress. From Pexels License. [Image]. https://www.pexels.com/photo/person-in-white-shirt-with-brown-wooden-frame-4769486/

Denton, C. (2016). What Do Specific Foods Do? | Taking Charge of Your Health & Wellbeing. Taking Charge of Your Health & Wellbeing. https://www.takingcharge.csh.umn.edu/explore-healing-practices/food-medicine/what-do-specific-foods-do

Denton, C. (2019). How Does Food Impact Health? | Taking Charge of Your Health &

AFTERWORD

Wellbeing. Taking Charge of Your Health & Wellbeing. https://www.takingcharge.csh.umn.edu/how-does-food-impact-health

DiGiulio, S. (2017). What Happens in Your Body and Brain While You Sleep. NBC News; NBC News. https://www.nbcnews.com/better/health/what-happens-your-body-brain-while-you-sleep-ncna805276

Dogra, T. (2020). 5 Aspects of Holistic Health: Know Why They Are So Important? Onlymyhealth. https://www.onlymyhealth.com/know-why-aspects-of-holistic-health-are-important-1594372951

Du Preez, P. (2017). Music. From Unsplash License. [Image]. https://unsplash.com/photos/XZEYdvJznMQ

Earle, J. (2016). Nature. From Unsplash License. [Image]. https://unsplash.com/photos/ICE__bo2Vws

Friedman, L. T. (2021). Signs Of a Clogged Lymphatic System & 10 Ways to Cleanse It | eshrh. Synergyhealthassociates.com. https://synergyhealthassociates.com/blog/cleanse-clogged-lymphatic-system

Gomes, C. (2018). Health & Wellness. From Unsplash License. [Image]. https://unsplash.com/photos/QDq3YliZg48

AFTERWORD

Goodson, A. (2018). The 19 Best Foods to Improve Digestion. Healthline. https://www.healthline.com/nutrition/best-foods-for-digestion#TOC_TITLE_HDR_8

Gorse, M. (2019). 9 Foods to Naturally Detox - Patient First. Www.patientfirst.com. https://www.patientfirst.com/blog/9-foods-to-naturally-detox

Holistic Healing: Six Steps to Holistic Health. (2016). Healthy Hildegard. https://www.healthyhildegard.com/holistic-healing/

Jones, T. (2021). Does Food Combining Work? Fact or Fiction. Healthline. https://www.healthline.com/nutrition/food-combining#TOC_TITLE_HDR_2

KnowYourOTCS. (2019). Dietary Supplements: Make Sure You Get the Benefits. https://www.knowyourotcs.org/dietary-supplements-make-sure-get-benefits

Kolasa-Sikiaridi, K. (2021). 10 Little-Known Natural Home Remedies from Ancient Greece. GreekReporter.com. https://greekreporter.com/2021/05/28/10-little-known-natural-home-remedies-from-ancient-greece/

Kubala, J. (2018a). The 14 Best Foods to

AFTERWORD

Increase Blood Flow and Circulation. Healthline; Healthline Media. https://www.healthline.com/nutrition/foods-that-increase-blood-flow

Kubala, J. (2018b). The 14 Best Foods to Increase Blood Flow and Circulation. Healthline; Healthline Media. https://www.healthline.com/nutrition/foods-that-increase-blood-flow

Kubala, J. (2018c). The 25 Best Diet Tips to Lose Weight and Improve Health. Healthline; Healthline Media. https://www.healthline.com/nutrition/25-best-diet-tips

Kubala, J. (2020a). The 20 Best Foods for Lung Health. Healthline. https://www.healthline.com/nutrition/lung-cleansing-foods#1.-Beets-and-beet-greens

Kubala, J. (2020b). The 20 Best Foods for Lung Health. Healthline. https://www.healthline.com/nutrition/lung-cleansing-foods#1.-Beets-and-beet-greens

L.Ac, C. (2016). How To Heal Yourself from The Inside Out. Sophia Natural Health. https://inm.center/heal-yourself/

Lark, B. (2017a). Food Combining. From Unsplash License. [Image]. https://unsplash.com/photos/V4MBq8kue3U

Lark, B. (2017b). Nutrition. From Unsplash License. [Image]. https://unsplash.com/photos/jUPOXXRNdcA

Leech, J. (2018). The Alkaline Diet: An Evidence-Based Review. Healthline; Healthline Media. https://www.healthline.com/nutrition/the-alkaline-diet-myth

Lopes, H. (2017). Friends. From Unsplash License. [Image]. https://unsplash.com/photos/e3OUQGT9bWU

Lowery, M. (2019). The 80/20 Rule, What Is It and How to Apply It? 2mealday.com. https://2mealday.com/article/the-80-20-rule-what-is-it-and-how-to-apply-it/

Lund, M. (2013). Integrative Medicine Embraces Nutrition. Todaysdietitian.com. https://www.todaysdietitian.com/newarchives/021313p26.shtml

Lundquist, E. (2019). Is the body designed to heal itself? TCIM. https://www.tcimedicine.com/post/is-the-body-designed-to-heal-itself

Morris, S. (2019). Supplements for Holistic Health - Discover 7 Key Holistic Supplements. ZYTO. https://zyto.com/7-holistic-health-supplements

Nunez, K. (2020). Our Holistic Doctors

AFTERWORD

Real Doctors? The Principles of Holistic Medicine. Healthline. https://www.healthline.com/health/holistic-doctor#What-is-holistic-medicine?

Petre, A. (2018). 8 Common Signs of Vitamin Deficiency, Plus How to Fix Them. Healthline. https://www.healthline.com/nutrition/vitamin-deficiency

Ragland, L. (2020). Stress Management: Ways to Prevent and Relieve Stress. WebMD; WebMD. https://www.webmd.com/balance/stress-management/stress-management

Redl, A. (2017). Athletics. From Unsplash License. [Image]. https://unsplash.com/photos/d3bYmnZ0ank

Robertson, R. (2018). The Gut-Brain Connection: How it Works and The Role of Nutrition. Healthline. https://www.healthline.com/nutrition/gut-brain-connection#TOC_TITLE_HDR_2

Roger Williams University. (2019). Dimensions of Wellness | Roger Williams University. Rwu.edu. https://www.rwu.edu/undergraduate/student-life/health-and-counseling/health-education-program/dimensions-wellness

Schättin, A., Baur, K., Stutz, J., Wolf, P., &

de Bruin, E. D. (2016). Effects of Physical Exercise Combined with Nutritional Supplements on Aging Brain Related Structures and Functions: A Systematic Review. Front. Aging Neurosci. https://doi.org/https://doi.org/10.3389/fnagi.2016.00161

Shkraba, A. (2020). Acupuncture. From Pexels License. [Image]. https://www.pexels.com/photo/a-person-applying-acupuncture-needle-on-client-s-forehead-6076141/

Shvets, A. (2020). Dentition. From Pexels License. [Image]. https://www.pexels.com/photo/person-with-dental-cheek-retractor-3845856/

Slowikowska, V. (2020). Cooking. From Pexels License. [Image]. https://www.pexels.com/photo/person-slicing-a-vegetable-on-wooden-chopping-board-5677302/

Tankilevitch, P. (2020). Grains. From Pexels License. [Image]. https://www.pexels.com/photo/close-up-photo-of-rice-on-person-s-hand-4110256/

Taran, O. (2020). Exercise. From Unsplash License. [Image]. https://unsplash.com/photos/xB4ExGcUai0

Templeton, J. (2017). The 8 Pillars of

AFTERWORD

Holistic Health and Wellness. Ask the Scientists. https://askthescientists.com/pillars-of-wellness/

The 5 Aspects Of Holistic Health And Why They Are So Important. (2020). The Well Co. https://www.thewellessentials.com/blog/the-5-aspects-of-holistic-health-and-why-they-are-so-important/

The New York Public Library. (2019). Agriculture. From Unsplash License. [Image]. https://unsplash.com/photos/4xE-RVLLwTQ

Tountas, Y. (2017). The Roots of Holistic Health. Greece Is. https://www.greece-is.com/the-roots-of-holistic-health/

Tuunainen, R. (2017). Supplement. From Pixabay License. [Image]. https://pixabay.com/photos/medicine-capsule-blue-white-2207622/

Волк, М. (2020). Alkaline Drink. From Unsplash License. [Image]. https://unsplash.com/photos/7O-__rhcZ5Y

World Health Organization (WHO)). (2022). Healthy diet. Www.who.int. https://www.who.int/health-topics/healthy-diet#tab=tab_2

Xo, K. (2017). Holistic Nutrition: A Beginner's Guide. The Wholesome Witch.

AFTERWORD

https://www.thewholesomewitch.com/holistic-nutrition-beginners-guide/

Your Body's Systems. (2017). Fact Monster. https://www.factmonster.com/math-science/biology/human-body/your-bodys-systems#:~:text=Your%20Body%27s%20Systems%201%20Circulatory%20System.%20The%20circulatory

ABOUT THE AUTHOR

Yota Kouyas Gerrior R.H.N is an emerging author of Holisitc Health & Wellness Practices. For ten years, Yota has been researching and studying ways to improve her overall health. After studying at CSNN, The Canadian School of Natural Nutrition, she decided to start a series of books to share her findings with others; in hopes that she can help others find ways to improve their overall health and wellness. If you liked this book, you might also be interested in her second book on Amazon called "The Holistic Greek Diet & Way of Life". You can also join Yota's Holisitc Health and Wellness Practices Community on Facebook and Instagram.

ALSO BY
YOTA KOUYAS GERRIOR R.H.N

The Holistic Greek Diet & Way of Life

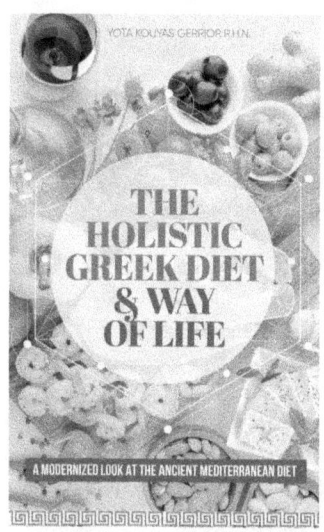

A Modernised Look at the Ancient Mediterranean Diet

To sign up for Yota's mailing list and her Holisitc Health and Wellness Practices visit link below:

www.yotasholistichealth.com

www.ingramcontent.com/pod-product-compliance
Lightning Source LLC
Chambersburg PA
CBHW020254030426
42336CB00010B/755